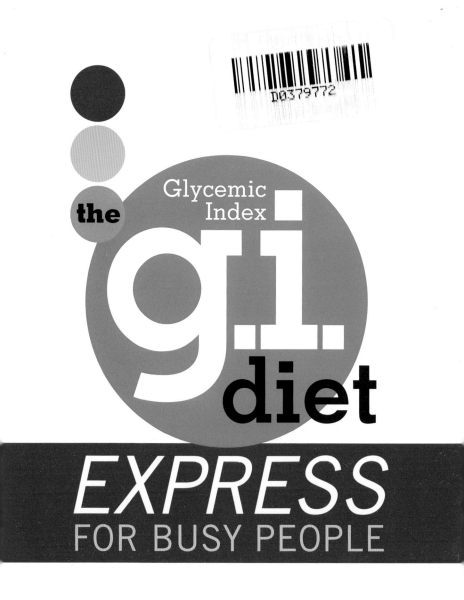

the **g.i.** diet

Glycemic Index

EXPRESS
FOR BUSY PEOPLE

D0379772

First published in the United States in 2007 by

Virgin Books Ltd

Thames Wharf Studios

Rainville Road

London

W6 9HA

Copyright © 2007 Green Light Foods Inc.

By arrangement with Westwood Creative Artists Ltd.

Distributed by Holtzbrinck Publishers.

A catalogue record for this book is available from the British Library.

ISBN 978 0 7535 1183 1

Designed & Typeset by Virgin Books Ltd

Printed and bound in Italy

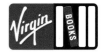

the
Glycemic
Index
g.i. diet

EXPRESS
FOR BUSY PEOPLE

With 50 speedy recipes

RICK GALLOP

Contents

INTRODUCTION   7

CHAPTER 1: THE G.I. DIET IN A NUTSHELL   10

CHAPTER 2: GETTING STARTED   17

CHAPTER 3: GREEN LIGHT SHOPPING   24

CHAPTER 4: INTRODUCTION TO GREEN LIGHT COOKING   46

CHAPTER 5: PHASE ONE—LOSING WEIGHT   56

CHAPTER 6: PHASE TWO—HOW YOU WILL EAT
FOR THE REST OF YOUR LIFE   123

CHAPTER 7: TOP FIVE FAQS
(FREQUENTLY ASKED QUESTIONS)   125

CHAPTER 8: EXERCISE   128

APPENDIX I: COMPLETE G.I. DIET FOOD GUIDE   130

APPENDIX II: SEVEN-DAY MEAL PLAN   144

APPENDIX III: WEEKLY WEIGHT AND WAIST LOG   152

APPENDIX IV: G.I. DIET READERS' LETTERS   154

INDEX   156

Introduction

Since the launch of my first book, *The G.I. Diet*, four years ago, some two million books have been sold worldwide. The reasons for its success are simple

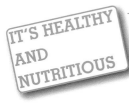

Hundreds of thousands of people have lost weight permanently and painlessly without going hungry or feeling deprived.

There's no counting calories or points. No weighing and measuring foods. All foods are traffic-light color-coded, so just follow the green lights.

Unlike many diets, it's a healthy, balanced diet that will guide you for the rest of your life.

I've also received, to my surprise, a flood of over 25,000 e-mails from readers. From these e-mails I've learned a great deal about the real-world challenges people face when trying to change their lifestyle and diet. Many of the responses focused on a need for more recipes which resulted in a new cookbook—*Living the G.I. Diet*. Recently I've been hearing more and more about time pressures and have been getting questions on how to manage the G.I. Diet on a busy schedule. With demanding jobs, busy family lives and the fact that there are simply not enough hours in the day, many of you admit to letting matters of health and weight take a back seat.

The G.I. Diet Express is designed to address the challenges of permanently changing the way you eat while living in today's hectic world. It provides practical hands-on advice on shopping and stocking the pantry with the right green light essentials; suggestions for on-the-run and sit-down breakfasts; brown-bag lunches and eating out in fast-food restaurants; plus dozens of delicious dinner recipes and lots of tasty snacks to help keep you going. All food is quick and easy to prepare.

I've also included some advice on exercise and how to incorporate it into your busy day.

> ## "The G.I. Diet Express means you'll never be too busy to lose weight!"

My wife, Dr Ruth Gallop, has been my partner for 35 years and has during that time taken on executive responsibility for nutrition and health in our household of three boys. She has written most of the sections on food preparation and recipes in conjunction with her close friend and food expert Natalie Stein. We've also had the advice and counsel of one of our country's brilliant young cooks, Laura Buckley.

You no longer have the excuse that you are too busy to be managing your weight and looking after your health. *The G.I. Diet Express* builds on the hugely successful G.I. Diet, which has changed the lives of literally tens of thousands of readers, by adapting it to meet the needs of your busy life.

If you are interested in receiving the free quarterly G.I. Diet Newsletter, go to www.gidiet.com and sign up. The website also features readers' comments, medical and media reviews, and reports on new developments in health and nutrition. You can also contact me through this website—I'd love to hear about your experiences, along with your comments and suggestions. Enjoy!

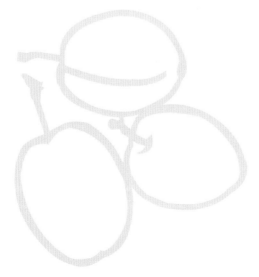

Chapter 1: The G.I. Diet in a Nutshell

G.I. stands for Glycemic Index, a medical term used to measure the speed at which carbohydrates break down in the digestive system to form glucose (sugar). Glucose is the body's source of energy—it is the fuel that feeds your brain, muscles, and other organs. Sugar is set at 100, and all foods are indexed against that number. So foods that are quickly digested have a high G.I. and foods that are digested more slowly have a lower G.I. Here are some popular examples, showing high G.I. foods in the left column and low G.I. in the right.

EXAMPLES OF G.I. RATINGS

High G.I.		Low G.I.*	
Foods	Rating	Foods	Rating
Sugar	100	Orange	44
Baguette	95	All Bran	43
Cornflakes	84	Oatmeal	42
Rice cakes	82	Spaghetti	41
Donut	76	Apples	38
Bagel	72	Beans	31
Cereal bar	72	Grapefruit	25
Cookies (plain)	69	Yogurt	14

* Any food rating less than 55 in the G.I. is considered low

So what's this got to do with losing weight? Lots! When you eat high G.I. foods, such as cornflakes, your body rapidly converts them into glucose, which dissolves in your bloodstream, spiking your blood-sugar level and giving you that familiar sugar rush or high. But when you eat a low G.I. food, such as oatmeal, it will break down more slowly and deliver the glucose into the bloodstream at a slower but steady rate.

"Low G.I. foods are digested slowly, high G.I. foods are digested quickly"

The following chart demonstrates the different impact of high and low G.I. foods on your blood-sugar levels.

G.I. IMPACT ON SUGAR LEVELS

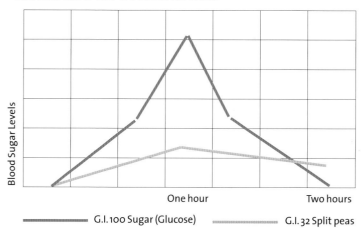

Blood Sugar Levels

One hour   Two hours

▬▬▬▬▬ G.I. 100 Sugar (Glucose)   ▬▬▬▬▬ G.I. 32 Split peas

The sugar spike is short-lived, however, because of a critical enzyme called insulin, whose job is to take sugar from the bloodstream and store it for immediate use in your muscles or as fat around your waist, hips, and thighs. The higher the sugar spike, the more insulin is released, and the quicker the sugar is drained from your bloodstream, leaving you with a sugar low. And we all know what happens then—you start looking for your next quick sugar fix. That is why after your high G.I. breakfast of sugary cold cereal, you are reaching for a Danish and coffee as soon as you reach the office. So a diet of high G.I. foods obviously makes you feel hungry more often, which means you will end up eating more.

Conversely, low G.I. foods, because they break down more slowly, deliver a steady stream of glucose and do not trigger a sugar spike or a flood of insulin. As a result, you feel fuller for a longer period of time and therefore eat less without going hungry. And eating less without going hungry or feeling deprived is the key to any successful diet.

"Low G.I. foods leave you feeling fuller for longer, so you won't go craving that sugar fix"

These sugars or carbs (carbohydrates) account for over half of our energy needs. But we also have two other critical food groups to consider, namely proteins and fats.

Proteins are essential for our health. Half of our dry body weight is made up of protein, including our muscles, organs, skin, and hair. Protein is required to build and repair body tissue, and is also very effective at satisfying hunger, as it acts as a brake on the digestive system. So, like low G.I. carbs, protein helps you feel fuller for a longer period. Unfortunately, much of our protein comes from animal sources, which are usually high in saturated or "bad" fat. So lean protein found in lean meats, fish, poultry, and soy are your best green light choices.

Fat is also essential for our health and our bodily functions. However, many fats are positively dangerous to your health and can increase your risk of heart disease, stroke, and some cancers. These fats are called saturated fats and are normally solid at room temperature, e.g. cheese, butter, and fatty meats. Even worse are trans fats or hydrogenated fats, which have been processed to make them thicken. These are often found in store-bought crackers, chips, and other snacks. Your best choices are polyunsaturated fats—most vegetable oils fall into this category. Even better are monounsaturated fats, such as olive, canola, peanut, and safflower oils, and most nuts—particularly almonds. A special oil called omega-3, found in deep-sea fish such as salmon, as well as in flaxseed, is great for your heart health.

As fats have more than twice the calories per gram as carbs and proteins, you must be careful of the quantity of fat you consume.

So the ideal combination of foods is low G.I. carbohydrates, lean protein, and monounsaturated/polyunsaturated fats.

TRAFFIC LIGHTS

To keep things simple so you don't have to worry about calculating G.I. ratings, calorie counts, and saturated fat levels, we have done all the math for you. The results have been color-coded into three traffic-light colors.

"The traffic-light system means no more counting calories or points"

RED LIGHT FOODS

Do not eat these foods if you want to lose weight. These are both higher G.I. and higher calorie foods.

YELLOW LIGHT FOODS

Eat only once you have reached your target weight. These are the mid-range G.I. foods.

GREENLIGHT FOODS

With a few exceptions (see below), you can eat as much of these foods as you like. Remember, everything in moderation! These foods are low G.I., low in calories, and low in saturated (bad) fat.

RECOMMENDED GREEN-LIGHT SERVINGS

Greenlight breads (at least 2½–3g of fiber per slice)	1 slice
Greenlight cereals	1/2 cup
Greenlight nuts	8 to 10 (small handful)
Margarine (non-hydrogenated, light)	2 teaspoons
Meat, fish, poultry	4oz (the size of a pack of cards)
Olive/vegetable oil	1 teaspoon
Olives	4 to 5
Pasta	3/4 cup cooked
Potatoes (new, boiled)	2 to 3
Rice (basmati, brown, long-grain)	2/3 cup cooked
Phase II	
Chocolate (at least 70% cocoa)	2 squares
Red wine	1 glass (5 ounces)

MEALS

We strongly recommend eating three main meals and three snacks between meals; mid-morning, mid-afternoon, and before bed. The important thing is to keep your blood-sugar levels constant and avoid the sugar highs and lows, which is the usual reason people overeat. Keeping your tummy busy and your blood-sugar levels constant is fundamental to the success of the G.I. Diet.

PORTIONS

Each meal and snack should contain a combination of green light carbohydrates, protein, and fats. An easy way to visualize your dinner plate is to divide it into three sections—half your plate should be filled with vegetables, a quarter with meat/fish/poultry/tofu, and the remaining quarter with rice/pasta/potatoes.

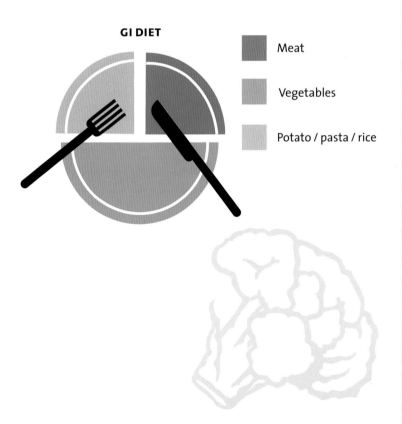

GI DIET

Meat

Vegetables

Potato / pasta / rice

TIMING

There are two phases to the G.I. Diet.

PHASE ONE—THE WEIGHT LOSS PHASE

During this phase you should eat green light foods only. You should lose an average of one pound per week. If you have a significant amount of weight to lose, then you should lose two pounds or more per week.

PHASE TWO—THE MAINTENANCE PHASE

Once you have reached your target weight you can include yellow light foods. This is how you will eat for the rest of your life.

SUMMARY

- Low G.I. foods are slower to digest, so you feel satisfied for longer
- Green light foods are key to losing weight as they are low G.I., low in calories and low in saturated fats
- During Phase One, eat only green light foods
- Eat three balanced meals and three snacks per day

Chapter 2: Getting Started

There are three simple steps to getting started on the Express G.I. Diet.

● **Set your weight loss target**

● Clear out your pantry/refrigerator

● Go green light shopping

WEIGHT-LOSS TARGET

Although how much weight you want to lose is strictly a personal decision, here are some guidelines that might help.

BODY MASS INDEX (BMI)

BMI is the only internationally accepted measurement for assessing how much body fat you are carrying relative to your height. In the BMI table on page 18–19 simply find your height in the horizontal line across the top and go down the vertical line on the left to your current weight. Where the two columns intersect is your BMI.

BMI TABLE

WEIGHT	HEIGHT																		
FT INS	4'6"	4'8"	4'10"	5'0"	5'2"	5'3"	5'4"	5'5"	5'6"	5'7"	5'8"	5'9"	5'10"	5'11"	6'0"	6'2"	6'4"	6'6"	6'8"
POUNDS																			
91	22.0	20.4	19.0	17.8	16.6	16.1	15.6	15.1	14.7	14.3	13.8	13.4	13.1	12.7	12.3	11.7	11.1	10.5	10.0
94	22.7	21.1	19.6	18.4	17.2	16.7	16.1	15.6	15.2	14.7	14.3	13.9	13.5	13.1	12.7	12.1	11.4	10.9	10.3
98	23.7	22.0	20.5	19.1	17.9	17.4	16.8	16.3	15.8	15.3	14.9	14.5	14.1	13.7	13.3	12.6	11.9	11.3	10.8
101	24.4	22.6	21.1	19.7	18.5	17.9	17.3	16.8	16.3	15.8	15.4	14.9	14.5	14.1	13.7	13.0	12.3	11.7	11.1
105	25.4	23.5	21.9	20.5	19.2	18.6	18.0	17.5	16.9	16.4	16.0	15.5	15.1	14.6	14.2	13.5	12.8	12.1	11.5
108	26.1	24.2	22.6	21.1	19.8	19.1	18.5	18.0	17.4	16.9	16.4	15.9	15.5	15.1	14.6	13.9	13.1	12.5	11.9
112	27.1	25.1	23.4	21.9	20.5	19.8	19.2	18.6	18.1	17.5	17.0	16.5	16.1	15.6	15.2	14.4	13.6	12.9	12.3
115	27.8	25.8	24.0	22.5	21.0	20.4	19.7	19.1	18.6	18.0	17.5	17.0	16.5	16.0	15.6	14.8	14.0	13.3	12.6
119	28.8	26.7	24.9	23.2	21.8	21.1	20.4	19.8	19.2	18.6	18.1	17.6	17.1	16.6	16.1	15.3	14.5	13.8	13.1
122	29.5	27.4	25.5	23.8	22.3	21.6	20.9	20.3	19.7	19.1	18.5	18.0	17.5	17.0	16.5	15.7	14.9	14.1	13.4
129	31.2	28.9	27.0	25.2	23.6	22.9	22.1	21.5	20.8	20.2	19.6	19.0	18.5	18.0	17.5	16.6	15.7	14.9	14.2
133	32.1	29.8	27.8	26.0	24.3	23.6	22.8	22.1	21.5	20.8	20.2	19.6	19.1	18.5	18.0	17.1	16.2	15.4	14.6
136	32.9	30.5	28.4	26.6	24.9	24.1	23.3	22.6	22.0	21.3	20.7	20.1	19.5	19.0	18.4	17.5	16.6	15.7	14.9
140	33.8	31.4	29.3	27.3	25.6	24.8	24.0	23.3	22.6	21.9	21.3	20.7	20.1	19.5	19.0	18.0	17.0	16.2	15.4
143	34.6	32.1	29.9	27.9	26.2	25.3	24.5	23.8	23.1	22.4	21.7	21.1	20.5	19.9	19.4	18.4	17.4	16.5	15.7
147	35.5	33.0	30.7	28.7	26.9	26.0	25.2	24.5	23.7	23.0	22.4	21.7	21.1	20.5	19.9	18.9	17.9	17.0	16.1
150	36.3	33.6	31.3	29.3	27.4	26.6	25.7	25.0	24.2	23.5	22.8	22.2	21.5	20.9	20.3	19.3	18.3	17.3	16.5
154	37.2	34.5	32.2	30.1	28.2	27.3	26.4	25.6	24.9	24.1	23.4	22.7	22.1	21.5	20.9	19.8	18.7	17.8	16.9
157	37.9	35.2	32.8	30.7	28.7	27.8	26.9	26.1	25.3	24.6	23.9	23.2	22.5	21.9	21.3	20.2	19.1	18.1	17.2
161	38.9	36.1	33.6	31.4	29.4	28.5	27.6	26.8	26.0	25.2	24.5	23.8	23.1	22.5	21.8	20.7	19.6	18.6	17.7
164	39.6	36.8	34.3	32.0	30.0	29.1	28.2	27.3	26.5	25.7	24.9	24.2	23.5	22.9	22.2	21.1	20.0	19.0	18.0
168	40.6	37.7	35.1	32.8	30.7	29.8	28.8	28.0	27.1	26.3	25.5	24.8	24.1	23.4	22.8	21.6	20.4	19.4	18.5
171	41.3	38.3	35.7	33.4	31.3	30.3	29.4	28.5	27.6	26.8	26.0	25.3	24.5	23.8	23.2	22.0	20.8	19.8	18.8
175	42.3	39.2	36.6	34.2	32.0	31.0	30.0	29.1	28.2	27.4	26.6	25.8	25.1	24.4	23.7	22.5	21.3	20.2	19.2

178	43.0	39.9	37.2	34.8	32.6	31.5	30.6	29.6	28.7	27.9	27.1	26.3	25.5	24.8	24.1	22.9	21.7	20.6	19.6
182	44.0	40.8	38.0	35.5	33.3	32.2	31.2	30.3	29.4	28.5	27.7	26.9	26.1	25.4	24.7	23.4	22.2	21.0	20.0
185	44.7	41.5	38.7	36.1	33.8	32.8	31.8	30.8	29.9	29.0	28.1	27.3	26.5	25.8	25.1	23.8	22.5	21.4	20.3
189	45.7	42.4	39.5	36.9	34.6	33.5	32.4	31.5	30.5	29.6	28.7	27.9	27.1	26.4	25.6	24.3	23.0	21.8	20.8
192	46.4	43.0	40.1	37.5	35.1	34.0	33.0	31.9	31.0	30.1	29.2	28.4	27.5	26.8	26.0	24.7	23.4	22.2	21.1
196	47.4	43.9	41.0	38.3	35.8	34.7	33.6	32.6	31.6	30.7	29.8	28.9	28.1	27.3	26.6	25.2	23.9	22.6	21.5
199	48.1	44.6	41.6	38.9	36.4	35.3	34.2	33.1	32.1	31.2	30.3	29.4	28.6	27.8	27.0	25.5	24.2	23.0	21.9
203	49.1	45.5	42.4	39.6	37.1	36.0	34.8	33.8	32.8	31.8	30.9	30.0	29.1	28.3	27.5	26.1	24.7	23.5	22.3
206	49.8	46.2	43.1	40.2	37.7	36.5	35.4	34.3	33.2	32.3	31.3	30.4	29.6	28.7	27.9	26.4	25.1	23.8	22.6
210	50.8	47.1	43.9	41.0	38.4	37.2	36.0	34.9	33.9	32.9	31.9	31.0	30.1	29.3	28.5	27.0	25.6	24.3	23.1
213	51.5	47.8	44.5	41.6	39.0	37.7	36.6	35.4	34.4	33.4	32.4	31.5	30.6	29.7	28.9	27.3	25.9	24.6	23.4
217	52.4	48.6	45.4	42.4	39.7	38.4	37.2	36.1	35.0	34.0	33.0	32.0	31.1	30.3	29.4	27.9	26.4	25.1	23.8
220	53.2	49.3	46.0	43.0	40.2	39.0	37.8	36.6	35.5	34.5	33.5	32.5	31.6	30.7	29.8	28.2	26.8	25.4	24.2
224	54.1	50.2	46.8	43.7	41.0	39.7	38.4	37.3	36.2	35.1	34.1	33.1	32.1	31.2	30.4	28.8	27.3	25.9	24.6
227	54.9	50.9	47.4	44.3	41.5	40.2	39.0	37.8	36.6	35.6	34.5	33.5	32.6	31.7	30.8	29.1	27.6	26.2	24.9
231	55.8	51.8	48.3	45.1	42.2	40.9	39.7	38.4	37.3	36.2	35.1	34.1	33.1	32.2	31.3	29.7	28.1	26.7	25.4
234	56.6	52.5	48.9	45.7	42.8	41.5	40.2	38.9	37.8	36.6	35.6	34.6	33.6	32.6	31.7	30.0	28.5	27.0	25.7
238	57.5	53.4	49.7	46.5	43.5	42.2	40.9	39.6	38.4	37.3	36.2	35.1	34.1	33.2	32.2	30.6	29.0	27.5	26.1
245	59.0	54.9	51.2	47.8	44.8	43.3	42.0	40.7	39.5	38.3	37.2	36.1	35.1	34.1	33.2	31.4	29.8	28.3	26.9
252	60.7	56.4	52.6	49.2	46.0	44.6	43.2	41.9	40.6	39.4	38.3	37.2	36.1	35.1	34.1	32.3	30.5	29.1	27.6
259	62.4	58.0	54.1	50.5	47.3	45.8	44.4	43.0	41.8	40.5	39.3	38.2	37.1	36.1	35.1	33.2	31.5	29.9	28.4
266	64.1	59.6	55.5	51.9	48.6	47.1	45.6	44.2	42.9	41.6	40.4	39.2	38.1	37.0	36.0	34.1	32.3	30.7	29.2

Now check your results against the following BMI standards:

BMI rating	Indications
19–24	Healthy weight
25–29	Overweight
30–39	Obese
40 plus	Morbidly obese

Although these ratings apply to most people, those who have a large or small frame, or who are very muscular, may not fall into these ranges.

WAIST MEASUREMENT

Another guide to a healthy weight is where you carry this extra weight. Recent research has shown that belly fat represents the greatest risk to health.

People who carry their surplus weight around the middle are described as "apple-shaped", which is riskier to your health than carrying it around your hips—described as "pear-shaped". So check out your waistline (measured at the navel) against the following guidelines:

Healthy	Some Health Risk	Serious Health Risk
Women		
under 35 inches	35–37 inches	over 37 inches
Men		
under 37 inches	37–40 inches	over 40 inches

WAIST-TO-HIP MEASUREMENT

Though any surplus weight is potentially bad for your health, it is where you carry it that counts. Another way of looking at apple- versus pear-shaped is the waist-to-hip ratio. This is calculated by dividing your waist measurement by your hip measurement (i.e., the widest part of your butt). Check how you measure up against the standards.

Women: 0.8 or under (i.e. waist is 80% or less of hip measurement) is a healthy ratio.

Men: 0.95 or under (i.e. waist is 95% or less of hip measurement) is a healthy ratio.

These measurements—BMI, waist, and waist-to-hip ratio—will help you set your weight-loss targets.

TIMELINES

One of the most common questions I am asked is, "How long will it take to reach my target weight?"

As mentioned above, generally you should lose an average of one pound per week; if you are considerably overweight, this may well increase to an average of two pounds per week or more.

It is important to note that weight loss rarely occurs in a straight line but rather in a series of plateaus or steps. So don't panic if nothing happens for a week or two. Wait for your body to adjust and those pounds will come off.

Also, only weigh yourself weekly, on the same day at the same time of day. On getting up before breakfast is best (a meal or bowel movement can make a difference of a pound or more).

"Once your body adjusts to the diet the pounds will literally start to drop off!"

CLEAR OUT YOUR PANTRY/REFRIGERATOR

Before you go shopping for your green light foods, it is important to clear the decks and toss out those red light foods you will not be using again. If you are worried about waste, simply give the foods to charity or to your skinny neighbors!

Check the red light food listings on page 130.

This will remove temptation and if you have a partner or family, it sends a clear signal that things are going to change!

GREEN LIGHT SHOPPING

Before going shopping, make sure you don't go on an empty stomach or you could finish up with those tempting ready-to-eat red light foods at the checkout counter.

The next chapter of the book has been organized by supermarket department or aisle, such as fruit and vegetable aisle, deli counter, bakery, etc., so you can quickly identify where to find your favorite green light foods.

Because it would be impossible to list every brand in today's huge supermarkets, we have elected to list food categories, so for instance we list "Oatmeal", not "Quaker Oats". In a few instances, when there is clearly a "Best Buy", we do list the brand name.

However, in today's competitive marketplace most brands in any given category have similar formulations, so your choice will usually be made on quality and taste. In a few instances, where there may be some variations in content between brands—bread is a good example—you may want to check out the nutritional labels. Here is a typical label:

Nutrition Facts

Serving Size 1 cup (236ml)
Servings Per Container 1

Amount Per Serving

Calories 80   Calories from Fat 0

% Daily Value*

Total Fat 0g	0%
Saturated Fat 0g	0%
Trans Fat 0g	
Cholesterol Less than 5mg	0%
Sodium 120mg	5%
Total Carbohydtrate 11g	4%
Dietary Fiber 0g	0%
Sugars 11g	
Protien 9g	17%

Vitamin A 10%   •   Vitamin C 4%
Calcium 30% • Iron 0% • Vitamin D 25%

* Percent Daily Values are based on a 2,000
calorie diet. Your daily values may be higher or
lower depending on your calorie needs.

Serving Size: make sure you are comparing the same serving size

Calories: pick the lower calorie level

Fat: the lower the fat, especially saturated fat, the better

Salt: generally, the less the better

Fiber: higher is best, as it helps reduce the G.I.

Sugar: low, low, low

Protein: higher is better—protein helps slow digestion

SUMMARY
● Set weight/waist targets
● Clear the decks—pantry/refrigerator/freezer
● Go green-light shopping

Chapter 3: Green Light Shopping

This chapter consists of all the foods you will need for the basic meals and recipes in this book.

In each supermarket department, we list in **bold** those green light foods that are basic to the green light pantry and are commonly used in the recipes and meal suggestions in this book. This will help speed up your shopping. Other green light foods are used more occasionally—choosing them is very much a matter of your personal taste.

We have laid out the following section along the lines of the typical supermarket and have listed your best green light choices in each aisle, department, or counter. Writing a list will save you time and ensure that a key food doesn't get forgotten. Shopping the green light way will soon become second nature and a shopping list will probably become unnecessary.

A note on supermarket brands. Some supermarkets have made a real effort to improve the nutritional content of their house brands and are introducing new healthier choices that generally contain less sugar, saturated fats, and salt. This does not necessarily make them green light, but when in doubt about the best brand of choice in a given green light category, "healthy" brands are usually a best buy from a nutritional and price standpoint.

FRUIT AND VEGETABLE AISLE

VEGETABLES

These are the cornerstone of the G.I. Diet. They are low G.I. but high in fiber, and contain the nutrients, vitamins, and minerals that form the basis of a healthy and nutritious diet. Certain root vegetables are the exception to the rule.

As all cooking raises the G.I. and reduces nutritional content, always slightly undercook food, *al dente* as the Italians say, with some firmness to the bite. Microwaving in a little water is the recommended way to cook from both a speed and nutrition point of view. More on food preparation can be found in Cooking Basics, page 50.

Potatoes, along with rice, are the only principal foods that have different G.I. ratings depending on what type of potatoes you use and how you cook them. Large baked potatoes are high G.I. and therefore red light, as the baking process breaks down the fiber in them to make them more quickly digested. Small, preferably new, boiled potatoes have a far lower G.I. Don't mash them, as again this makes them digest more quickly.

Remember, the key to the G.I. Diet is slowing down the digestive process. We want your body—not the cooking—to do most of the processing. By the way, remember that frozen vegetables and fruits have the same G.I. rating and nutritional value as fresh.

Alfalfa sprouts
Arugula
Asparagus
Avocado
Beans (green/wax)
Bell peppers
Bok choy
Broccoli
Brussels sprouts
Cabbage (all varieties)
Capers
Carrots
Cauliflower
Celeriac
Celery

Collard greens
Cucumbers
Edamame (soybeans)
Eggplants
Endive
Escarole
Fresh herbs
Garlic
Ginger root
Green onions
Horseradish
Kale
Kohlrabi
Leeks
Lettuce (all varieties)
Mushrooms (all varieties)
Mustard greens
New potatoes
Okra
Olives
Onions
Peas
Pickles
Potatoes (boiled/new)
Radicchio
Radishes
Sauerkraut
Snow peas
Spinach
Sugar-snap peas
Sun-dried tomatoes
Swiss chard
Tomatoes
Watercress
Zucchinis

For a complete list of red, yellow and green light vegetables, see appendix 1 page 130.

FRUITS

Virtually all fresh/frozen fruits are low G.I. and green light. There are a few that are low in fiber and high in sugar, such as melons (including watermelons, which are high G.I. and therefore red light).

Fruits are an excellent source of fiber, vitamins, and minerals, all of which are essential for good health.

Apples
Blackberries
Blueberries
Cherries
Clementines
Cranberries
Grapefruit
Grapes
Guavas
Lemons
Mandarin oranges
Nectarines
Oranges
Peaches
Pears
Plums
Raspberries
Rhubarb
Strawberries
Tangerines

For a complete list of red, yellow and green light fruits see appendix 1 page 130.

THE DELI COUNTER

Most processed meats are high in saturated (bad) fat, salt, and nitrates and are therefore red light. Cheeses are generally loaded with saturated fat, though may be sprinkled on salads, omelets, and pasta for a little extra flavor. Lean processed meats and low-fat cheeses are your best green light options.

Chicken breast
Lean ham
Turkey breast

Cheese
Laughing Cow light
Boursin light
Fat-free cheese

Other
Olives
Hummus

For a complete list of red, yellow and green light deli counter products see appendix 1 page 130.

BAKERY

A word of warning about the bakery, as this can be a minefield of misinformation. Most baked foods, such as white bread, bagels, and croissants are made from white flour, meaning that all the nutrition, fiber, and essential oils have been stripped out of the original grain. This makes them easy to digest and results in a high G.I. rating—in other words, most baked goods are red light.

What we are looking for are baked goods made from 100 percent whole-wheat flour and whole grains. If the flour is stoneground, so much the better. With bread, we require at least 2½ to 3 grams of fiber per slice. Check your labels, because that apparently wholesome-looking seven-grain bread may well list as its principal ingredient unbleached or enriched white flour. The seven grains are mere decoration.

Crispbreads (high fiber)
100% stoneground wholewheat bread
Wholegrain high-fiber bread (2.5–3g of fiber per slice)

For a complete list of red, yellow and green light bakery products see appendix 1 page 130.

FISH COUNTER

All fish and shellfish are green light. Deep-sea fish such as salmon and cod are rich in omega-3 oils, which are great for heart and health. Fish should not be battered or breaded. Go to page 80 for the chance to savor many delicious seafood recipes. Remember, your serving size should be four ounces, or about the size of the palm of your hand.

Fish
All fresh fish
All frozen fish
Caviar
Fish canned in water
Pickled herring
Sashimi
Smoked fish
Squid

Shellfish
Clams (canned or fresh)
Crab (canned or fresh)
Lobster (canned or fresh)
Oysters (fresh or smoked)
Scallops
Scampi
Shrimps (canned or fresh)

For a complete list of red, yellow and green light fish and shellfish see appendix 1 page 130.

MEAT COUNTER

Most meats contain saturated fat. Some of this can be removed by trimming visible fat, but the rest is inherent in the meat. Therefore, it's important to select meats that are naturally lean, such as round or loin cuts. Skinless chicken or turkey breasts are the low-fat benchmark.

Other top non-meat choices, whether you are a vegetarian or not, are tofu and soy-based TVP (textured vegetable protein), which are low in saturated fat and high in protein. Again, remember your serving size must not exceed four ounces.

Beef
Extra-lean ground beef
Eye round
Top round

Pork
Canadian bacon
Lean ham
Tenderloin

Poultry
Chicken breast (skinless)
Turkey breast (skinless)

Veal
Cutlets
Loin chop
Rib roast
Shank

Other
Ostrich
Rabbit
Venison

Processed meats
Ham (deli style)
Pastrami (turkey)
Turkey breast
Turkey roll

For a complete list of red, yellow and green light meats see appendix 1 page 130.

CANNED BEANS/VEGETABLES AISLE

Beans/legumes are the perfect green light food, high in protein and fiber, yet low in fat. Unfortunately, canned beans have a higher G.I. than dried beans because of the high temperatures used in the canning process to avoid spoilage. They are, however, very convenient. Canned beans with added meat, sugar, or molasses should be avoided. It's always preferable to buy fresh or frozen vegetables rather than canned and is more efficient if you buy them in large family-sized packs.

Beans
Baked beans (low fat/low sugar)
Black beans
Black-eyed peas
Butter beans
Chickpeas
Italian beans
Kidney beans (red/white)
Lentils
Lima/butterbeans
Mung
Navy/haricot beans
Romano refried beans (low fat)
Soybeans
Split peas

Canned and bottled vegetables
Roasted red peppers
Canned tomatoes
Tomato purée

For a complete list of red, yellow and green light canned beans and vegetables see appendix 1 page 130.

PASTA AND SAUCES AISLE

Most pastas (other than canned) are green light, in particular whole-wheat versions. Always undercook (*al dente*, with some firmness to the bite). Serving size is important here. Use pasta as a side-dish starter, with a ¾-cup cooked serving, and not as the basis of your meal.

Choose sauces that are preferably low-sugar (light). Tomato sauce is rich in lycopene, which has been shown to reduce the risk of prostate cancer.

Pasta
Capellini
Cellophane noodles (mung bean)
Fettuccine
Linguine
Macaroni
Penne
Rigatoni
Spaghetti
Vermicelli

Pasta sauces
Light sauces with vegetables (no added sugar) e.g. Healthy
  Choice, Clasico

For a complete list of red, yellow and green light pastas and
pasta sauces see appendix 1 page 130.

CANNED SOUP AISLE

Canned foods have a higher G.I. rating than fresh or those
cooked from scratch, but they are very convenient when time is
limited. Soups are good fillers and help moderate the amount
you eat during the rest of the meal. Chunky vegetable soups
are the best choice, but avoid cream and puréed soups.

Soup
Bouillon (low sodium)
Chunky bean/vegetable e.g. Healthy Request
Miso soup

For a complete list of red, yellow and green light canned
soup see appendix 1 page 130.

GRAINS

Many whole grains, with all the nutrition and fiber intact, are green light. When it comes to rice, choose long-grain, as it has a much lower G.I. than sticky or glutinous short-grain rice (the sort found in Chinese restaurants or in Italian risotto rice).

Arrowroot flour
Barley
Buckwheat
Bulgur
Flaxseeds (ground)
Gram flour
Kamut (not puffed)
Long grain rice (basmati, wild, brown)
Quinoa
Wheat berries

For a complete list of red, yellow and green light grains see appendix 1 page 130.

INTERNATIONAL FOOD AISLE

There are many flavorful foods and sauces to choose from here. Experiment a little—you may surprise yourself!

Asian
Bamboo shoots (canned)
Buckwheat noodles
Cellophane (mung bean) noodles
Chili sauce
Curry paste
Dried seaweed
Hoisin sauce

Hot chili paste
Miso
Pickled ginger
Rice vinegar
Soy sauce (low sodium)
Teriyaki sauce
Wasabi
Water chestnuts (canned)

Mexican
Chipotle en adobo (jalapeno peppers in adobo sauce)
Green chilies (canned)
Pickled jalapenos
Salsa (no added sugar)
Taco sauce (no added sugar)

Middle Eastern
Falafel mix
Hummus
Tahini

For a complete list of red, yellow and green light
international foods see appendix 1 page 130.

OIL/VINEGAR/SALAD DRESSING/AISLE

Top choices for cooking oils are olive, canola, and flax.

Dressings should be low-fat. However, as acid slows
down the digestive process, thereby reducing the meal's
G.I., vinaigrettes are a best buy. Even better, make your own
vinaigrette just by mixing olive oil and balsamic vinegar.

Many condiments and pickles are low G.I. Check the labels
for those with sugar or other natural sweeteners, such as
ketchup and brown sauce, which are not recommended.

Cooking oil
Canola oil
Extra virgin olive oil
Flax oil
Olive oil
Safflower oil
Vegetable oil spray

Vinegar
Balsamic vinegar
Cider vinegar
Red wine vinegar
Rice vinegar
White vinegar
White wine vinegar

Salad dressings
Low-fat, low-sugar salad dressings
Low-fat, low-sugar vinaigrettes

Pickles
Capers
Cocktail onions
Dill pickles
Olives
Pickled hot peppers
Pickled mixed vegetables
Pickled mushrooms

Condiments
Chili sauce
Dijon mustard
Gravy mix (maximum 20 calories per ½ cup serving)
Horseradish
Hummus

Mayonnaise (fat free)
Mustard
Salsa (no added sugar)
Seafood sauce
Steak sauce
Tabasco
Teriyaki sauce
Worcestershire sauce

For a complete list of red, yellow and green light
condiments and dressings see appendix 1 page 130.

SNACKS AISLE

Snacks are an important part of the G.I. Diet, which
recommends three snacks per day. There are many red light
temptations here, so check the green light list below carefully,
in particular so-called "nutrition" or "meal-replacement" bars.
Most are cereal- and sugar-based and contain little nutritional
value. The ones to look for should contain at least 10 to 15
grams of protein and around 5 grams of fat per 50–60 gram
bar. Remember, half a bar per serving. Balance and Zone bars
are good green light choices.

Almonds
Applesauce (unsweetened)
Canned fruit salad
Canned mandarin oranges
Canned peaches in juice or water
Canned pears in juice or water
Cashews
Food bars (see above)
Hazelnuts
Macadamia nuts

Most fresh/frozen vegetables (see page 25)
Most fresh/forzen fruits (see page 27)
Pistachios
Salsa (no added sugar)
Seeds (most)
Soy nuts
Sugar-free hard candies
Sunflower seeds

For a complete list of red, yellow and green light snacks see appendix 1 page 130.

BAKING AISLE

While commercial baked goods are almost all red light, you can make your own sweet treats using the recipes on pages 117–121, as well as from my other books—*The G.I. Diet* and *Living the G.I. Diet*. End of commercial!

Although dried fruit is generally red or yellow light, a small amount is acceptable to add flavor to your baked dishes.

Splenda (sucralose) is derived from sugar but without the calories and is our preferred choice of sweetener.

Sweeteners
Aspartame
Equal
Splenda
Stevia
Sugar Twin
Sweet'N Low

Spices and flavorings
Bouillon (low sodium)
Broth (low sodium/low fat/chicken/beef/vegetable)

Chili powder
Extracts (vanilla, etc.)
Garlic
Herbs
Lemon juice
Pepper (fresh ground)
Salt
Seasoning mixes with no added sugar
Spices

Baking supplies
Almonds
Baking powder
Baking Soda
Cinnamon
Cashews
Cocoa
Hazelnuts
Macadamia nuts
Oat bran
Pumpkin seeds
Sunflower seeds
Vanilla extract
Wheat bran
Wheat germ
Wholewheat flour

For a complete list of red, yellow and green light baking products see appendix 1 page 130.

BREAKFAST FOODS

Most cold cereals have a high G.I. and are red light, as they are made principally from highly processed grains with the nutrition and fiber removed. These include so-called "natural" or "healthy" granola-type cereals, as they are high in sugar and low in fiber. Also avoid cereal bars (see Snacks, above).

Look for cold cereals that have at least **10 grams of fiber per serving**. They may not be much fun in themselves, but they can be dressed up with nuts, fruit, and yogurt.

The king of hot cereals is oatmeal made with large-flake traditional rolled oats (not instant or quick oats). It takes about three minutes to make in the microwave. Topped with fruit and nuts, this is absolutely my top choice for breakfast and something many of you will not have eaten since you were children. I receive more enthusiastic correspondence from readers about their rediscovery of oatmeal than any other single food!

Low-sugar or extra-fruit jams, where fruit is listed as the first ingredient, are terrific for whole-wheat toast or for flavoring cereals and low-fat dairy products such as yogurt and cottage cheese.

Cereal
100% bran
All-bran
Bran buds
Fiber 1
Fiber First
Kashi Go Lean
Large-flake oatmeal
Oat bran
Steel-cut oatmeal

Spreads and jams
Extra fruit, low sugar spread (fruit listed as first ingredient)

For a complete list of red, yellow and green light breakfast foods see appendix 1 page 130.

BEVERAGE AISLE

You need up to eight glasses of liquid a day to keep your body hydrated and healthy. We recommend a glass of water before every meal. Having your stomach partly filled with liquid makes you feel full more quickly, thus reducing the temptation to overeat.

Drinks containing caffeine tend to stimulate the appetite and are therefore red light. The exception is tea, which has far less caffeine than coffee. Tea is also a good source of flavanoids (antioxidants), which are beneficial for heart health. Decaf coffee is a good idea—the latest brands taste like the real thing.

With regards to fruit or vegetable juice, it is better to eat the original fruit or vegetable than drink the juice. The fruit or vegetable has a lower G.I., fewer calories, and more nutrients. An excellent choice is skim milk—try to drink a glass a day as a snack or in place of water at mealtimes. Light, plain soy milk is a great alternative.

Bottled water (sparkling or still)
Decaffeinated coffee
Diet soft drinks (without caffeine)
Herbal teas
Iced tea (with no added sugar)
Light instant chocolate
Tea (with or without caffeine)

For a complete list of red, yellow and green light beverages see appendix 1 page 130.

DAIRY AISLE

Low-fat dairy products are a G.I. Diet staple. They are rich in protein, calcium, and vitamin D. Regular or full-fat dairy foods are not recommended, as they are loaded with saturated fat, with butter and cheese among the principal villains. However, you can use small amounts of full-fat flavored cheeses as a flavor enhancer when sprinkled lightly on salads, omelets, and pasta. There are some excellent new ultra-low-fat cheeses that are acceptable.

Fruit-flavored, fat-free yogurts with sweetener are ideal for adding to breakfast cereals, as a snack, or as a topping for a fruit dessert. If you are lactose intolerant, soy milk is an increasingly popular choice. Look for plain, low-fat versions, as the flavored ones can contain high levels of sugar.

Milk
Buttermilk
Skim milk
Soy milk (plain, low-fat)

Cheese
Cheese (fat-free)
Cottage cheese (1% or fat-free)
Cream cheese (fat free)
Extra low-fat cheese (e.g. Laughing Cow light, Boursin light)
Low-fat soy cheese

Yogurt and sour cream
Frozen yogurt (low fat/no added sugar)
Fruit yogurt (fat free with sugar substitute)
Sour cream (fat free)

Butter and margarine
Soft margarine (nonhydrogenated light)

Eggs
Eggbeaters
Egg whites
Liquid eggs

For a complete list of red, yellow and green light dairy products see appendix 1 page 130.

FROZEN FOOD SECTION

Almost all the prepared meals found in the frozen food section of your supermarket are red light, because of the ingredients used and the way in which they are processed.

They are, however, very convenient, and if you are really pushed for time, you might want to keep a couple of prepared meals on hand for emergencies. Your best choices are the "healthy" brands. They are, however, usually light on vegetables, so always add a vegetable or two or a side salad.

The freezer section is a great source of convenient and time-saving green light foods. Frozen vegetables, fruit, and fish are all ideal green light choices. Just make sure vegetables aren't in a butter, cream, or cheese sauce and the fish is not battered or breaded. The family-size large packs of fruit and vegetables are a particularly good buy.

Vegetables
Asparagus
Beans (green/wax)
Bell peppers
Broccoli
Brussels sprouts
Carrots
Cauliflower
Okra
Peas
Spinach

Prepared foods
Chicken souvlaki
Extra-lean burgers
Frozen fish without breaded coating
Scallops and shrimps without breaded coating
Textured vegetable protein

Tofu
Veggie burgers

Desserts
Frozen soya desserts with less than 100 calories per ½
Ice cream (low-fat and no added sugar)

Fruit
Blackberries
Blueberries
Cherries
Cranberries
Mixed berries
Peaches
Raspberries
Rhubarb
Strawberries

For a complete list of red, yellow and green light frozen foods see appendix 1 page 130.

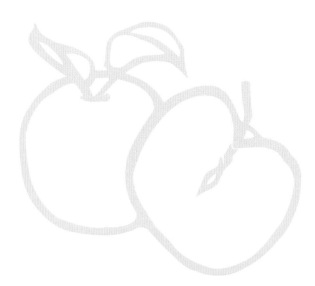

TIME SAVERS

Supermarkets have long recognized that many people have limited time to cook, and there is now an abundance of prepared and frozen foods available. With careful shopping, you can serve delicious green light meals with minimal effort.

All supermarkets carry the following:

- Precooked and sliced chicken breasts, often in various flavors but without sauce
- Prepared fish fillets or steaks, such as salmon—without sauce
- Prepared seafood, such as shrimp—without sauce, batter, or breading
- Packages of precut fresh vegetables, including mixed vegetables for stir-fries
- Packaged salad greens—many varieties

In the freezer look for:

- Sliced vegetables: many varieties are available, but avoid any in prepared sauces or butter
- Frozen fruits and berries

Most supermarkets also carry bottled garlic or garlic cubes for convenience. You can also find frozen fresh herbs and chopped ginger in some stores.

Chapter 4: Introduction to Green Light Cooking

The notion of going on a diet can be daunting. People are often fearful that their food choices will be limited to unappetizing, bland dishes that are tricky to prepare. This is definitely not the case with the G.I. Diet! You can eat very well on it and never have to sacrifice flavor or convenience. Not only are green light foods high in fiber and low in saturated fat and sugar, they are also some of the best-tasting foods around. Extra-virgin olive oil, for example, is a monounsaturated or "best" fat, which adds a wonderfully robust flavor to many dishes.

The key points with these recipes is that they are:

- Green light
- Easy and quick to prepare
- Delicious

Here are some tips on ingredients, equipment, and side dishes. You'll also find helpful advice on food preparation and cooking throughout the recipes.

INGREDIENTS

You will notice that not all the ingredients in the recipes are strictly green light. Occasionally I have added wine for depth of flavor as well as small amounts of sauces that contain sugar and dried fruit. This doesn't mean the recipe is yellow or red light. The quantities are small enough that they will have little or no effect on your blood-sugar levels, meaning they retain their green light status! To replace sugar in recipes, I use Splenda, a derivative of sugar but without the calories, with great success—the flavor is excellent. Look for the granular type because it is the easiest to use. Please note that all the major sugar substitutes used in cooking measure in equal volume to sugar. In other words, one tablespoon of sugar equals one tablespoon of sweetener.

SIDE DISHES
Almost all the dinner recipes I have included in this book should be accompanied by side dishes, especially salads. We have made "Sides Suggestions" in most recipes.

PORTIONS
Don't forget that a quarter of your plate should be filled with carbohydrates, such as pasta, rice, or boiled new potatoes. Since overcooking tends to raise the G.I. level of food, boil pasta until it is just *al dente*, and take rice off the heat before it starts to clump together. A quarter of your plate should contain lean protein—4 ounces (120 grams)—or enough to fit in the palm of your hand. The remaining half of your plate should be filled with green light vegetables and salads. Again, do not overcook the veggies; they should be tender-crisp. Who actually likes mushy vegetables, anyway?

RECIPE SERVINGS
Most of the recipes are devised for two persons, except where indicated.

THE EXPRESS KITCHEN
This book is written for busy people. You may be a working mom or dad rushing home after a day at work to rustle up dinner, or you could be a busy single person who has little time to cook. You could be a shift worker or a stay-at-home mom with small children demanding your full attention. Or maybe cooking is not a particularly pleasurable task for you but it has to be done. Whoever you are, you have decided to eat the healthy green light way but have little time to prepare meals.

The first thing to do is prepare the kitchen workspace. A little time spent doing this will reap enormous time-saving benefits as you prepare meals.

"The right equipment can save you valuable time in the kitchen."

THE EQUIPMENT

MICROWAVE OVEN

I believe microwave ovens were designed to make life easier. They have many more uses than reheating leftovers or thawing frozen meals, although both are useful functions. Fresh or frozen vegetables can be cooked in minutes and microwaving often preserves nutrients better than other methods because the cooking time is reduced and little water is used. When preparing vegetables, leave them in larger pieces, use small amounts of liquid, and cover to reduce cooking time. A serving of vegetables for two cooks to *al dente* in about three to five minutes. Fruit crumbles can be prepared in microwaves. They may not brown or crisp, but they will cook in a few minutes and still taste delicious.

OTHER USEFUL EQUIPMENT

- Measuring spoons
- Measuring cups for dry ingredients and liquids
- Good knives and a knife sharpener
- Nonstick skillets—have at least two of different sizes plus lids—really useful because it means you can cook with less oil and cleaning up is easy (you can apply oil with a light brush or use oil sprays)

- Steamer
- Tongs—plastic for the nonstick pans—make lifting, turning, and moving foods much easier
- Storage containers suitable for freezing
- Parchment paper—for lining trays in ovens—reduces clean-up time
- Grater—buy the kind that is flat in design and can be held over the pan or bowl so you can grate directly into the pot
- Cookbook holder

PLACING THE EQUIPMENT

Besides knowing where everything is, all your equipment should be at arm's reach of your cooking preparation site. This is true in both the small and large kitchen. Keep essentials on the counter if you have room so you don't have to pull them out each time you use them. Have wooden spoons, tongs, spatulas, etc. in a pot next to the stove. Herbs and spices should also be at arm's reach.

GETTING READY TO COOK

When you have chosen a recipe, get all your ingredients out at the beginning. Then have at hand the measuring cups and spoons, pots, and pans you will need. Do not start cooking before this. It wastes time to be running round the kitchen looking for food items and equipment.

COOKING BASICS FOR THE
EXPRESS G.I. DIET

BEANS AND LEGUMES

Beans and lentils are a great source of protein and fiber. For convenience, use canned beans. Just remember to rinse and drain thoroughly before use. Toss a handful of beans such as chickpeas, edamame (fresh soybeans), or kidney beans into your soup, salad, or stir-fry. Mixed beans tossed with chopped cucumber, tomato, red onion, parsley, or cilantro and dressing makes a tasty quick salad. Top with cooked chicken and lean ham and you have a meal.

FISH AND SEAFOOD

Fish and seafood can be quick and easy to prepare. Buy fish fresh, frozen or precooked. Just avoid fish that is breaded, fried, or in a sauce. The taste of a fillet is easily enhanced or varied by the addition of herbs, fruits, and other seasonings. If you don't have the time to prepare a topping, sprinkle on a small amount of dried herbes de Provence before cooking and top with a squeeze of lemon juice after.

In addition to sautéing, fish can be poached, steamed, baked, and grilled.

Approximate cooking times for four-ounce fillets are as follows:

Sauté uncovered:
Most fish can be sautéed. Season the fillet, then heat 1 teaspoon of oil in a nonstick skillet over a medium-high heat and cook for 2–3 minutes per side.

Sauté Covered:
This method keeps the fish very moist. Sauté uncovered for 1 minute per side as above. Then lower the heat, cover, and cook

until cooked through, about 4–5 minutes. The fish will feel firm to the touch and white juices will just start to appear.

Steamed:
Cook the fillets over boiling water for about 6–8 minutes. The fish will feel firm to the touch and white juices will just start to appear.

Grilled:
Fish can be cooked under a grill, on an outside barbecue, or in a grill pan. Spray the grill pan with oil, heat it, and grill the fish for 2–3 minutes per side. This method is great for salmon, tuna, and seafood such as shrimp.

Microwave:
Fish can be cooked quickly in a microwaveable dish. Cook covered in plastic wrap, leaving a small opening for steam, for about 5 minutes.

Note: It is important not to overcook fish. Cook until the flesh is opaque and firm but still moist. After a few tries you will know your stove or grill and the times required for each type of fish.

FRUIT
Fruit makes a great snack accompaniment or a sweet dessert. Use canned or frozen fruit (preferably frozen) when local fresh fruit is not available or too expensive. Remember to buy canned fruit in water or juice. If you do buy in syrup, drain and rinse the fruit before using. Thawed frozen raspberries or mixed berries with a little flavored yogurt make an easy dessert. Toss some frozen berries into your hot oatmeal or into your muffin mix for added flavor.

GARLIC

Buy one head at a time so the flavor stays fresh. Ready-to-use finely chopped garlic is available at the supermarket, either bottled or frozen.

GRAINS

Grains can be an excellent source of protein, fiber, and essential amino acids. Ground flaxseed can be sprinkled onto oatmeal or yogurt. While some grains such as barley take almost an hour to cook, grains such as quinoa and bulgur require less cooking time. Use in place of rice for a change in taste and texture.

HERBS AND SPICES

Herbs and spices are an essential element of flavorful cooking. For express cooking keep dried herbs and seasoning on hand. Buy them in small amounts and replace every three to six months. Do not keep them sitting by or on the stove—the heat will destroy their flavor.

Key herbs and spices include chili powder, cinnamon, cumin, ginger, basil, bay leaves, herbes de Provence, oregano, tarragon, and thyme.

PASTA

Use whole-wheat pasta where possible. For express cooking, put the pot of water plus a quarter of a teaspoon of salt on to boil as soon as you start the recipe. Use 1½ ounces of dry pasta per serving. Cook the pasta according to package directions until al dente.

POTATOES

Use two or three boiled new potatoes per serving. To save time, bring water to a boil at the beginning of the recipe. Small potatoes cook in approximately ten to twelve minutes. Season with chopped fresh parsley, a little lemon juice, and freshly ground pepper.

POULTRY

Skinless, boneless chicken breasts can be prepared quickly and with a minimum of fuss. They can be cooked whole or flattened as a cutlet. To make a cutlet, place a breast between plastic wrap and pound with a rolling pin or mallet until about 3/4 in. thick. Cut the breast or cutlet into strips or cubes for super-fast stir-fries. Always cook chicken until it is no longer pink inside and its juices run clear. For a whole breast (4 to 5 ounces) this usually means about six to eight minutes per side. Cutlets, strips, or cubes require less time.

Variety is the spice of life, as they say, and there is no reason your dishes can't be as varied and interesting as possible, with the help of easy-to-make sauces, salsas, and seasonings. We have provided plenty of suggestions for you. After you have cooked the chicken, simply use the pan juices as a base for sauces: add liquid and some seasoning, simmer for a few minutes, and serve!

RICE

Use long-grain basmati rice and rinse well before using. Bring water or broth to a boil at the beginning of the recipe, add the rice, cover, and simmer so the rice is ready when the main recipe has been cooked. Basmati rice takes about fifteen to twenty minutes to cook. Brown rice is an excellent choice too, but it takes longer to cook (around 30 to 45 minutes). If you want to use brown rice, factor in the added time—once it's on, you don't have to stir or fuss.

SALADS

Supermarkets sell a wide variety of salad greens ready to use—there's no need to get bored with the same old salad every day. Varieties include arugula, baby spinach, frisée, red-leaf lettuce, romaine, and watercress, to name a few. Add fresh tomatoes, sliced cucumber, and red onion for a traditional mixed salad. Try adding some beans, such as chickpeas, or other chopped fresh vegetables. Add sliced or chopped pear and a crumble of blue cheese with white-wine vinaigrette to baby spinach for a delicious salad. Other good additions to salad greens are strawberries, blueberries, raspberries, or chopped peaches or nectarines, tossed with a vinaigrette.

SALAD DRESSINGS

There are many low-fat, low-sugar dressings available. If you have time, make your own. Keep a variety of wine vinegars on hand as well as balsamic vinegar and mix with olive oil, Dijon mustard, and freshly ground pepper for basic vinaigrette variety. When you're in a real rush, just toss greens with balsamic vinegar and oil and freshly ground pepper.

SWEETENERS

Despite an intensive disinformation campaign by the sugar lobby, sugar substitutes are completely safe and approved by all major government and health authorities worldwide. If you are sensitive to aspartame, try one of the many alternatives.

The best form to use is granular, as it can be measured exactly the same as sugar by volume (not weight), meaning one tablespoon of sugar equals one tablespoon of sweetener. Our own preference is for Splenda, which is based on sucralose, and is ideal for baking.

VEGETABLES

The G.I. Diet places a lot of emphasis on vegetables, and half of your dinner plate should be made up of vegetables. You can use fresh or frozen vegetables—the nutrients are the same. Frozen vegetables are usually chopped or cut and ready for use, and supermarkets also sell prepared packages of vegetables ready for stir-fries or steaming, all of which will save you valuable time.

Vegetables can be prepared in many ways:

Microwave:
A microwave is a great time-saver. Cut the vegetables into serving pieces, add a small amount of water, cover, and cook on high. Two servings of most vegetables will cook in about 3–5 minutes. Cook until the vegetables are done but still crunchy.

Steaming:
Heat 1–2 inches of water in a large covered pot. Place the vegetables in a steamer basket and cover. Cook for a couple of minutes, checking the vegetables regularly to make sure they're still crunchy. This is a great method for asparagus, broccoli, green beans, and mixed vegetables.

Stir-fry:
Prepare the vegetables in bite-size or small pieces. Spray a nonstick wok or skillet with 1 teaspoon of vegetable oil or olive oil and heat. Stir-fry the vegetables for a couple of minutes, then add finely chopped garlic and/or ginger. Add a small amount of liquid, such as soy sauce or lemon juice, and continue cooking for a few minutes, until the vegetables are done. Toss in some cooked chicken, turkey, shrimp, firm tofu, or lean ham. This is a great method for cooking bell peppers, mushrooms, zucchini, sugar-snap peas, and snow peas.

Greens such as spinach, bok choy, baby bok choy, chard, kale, and broccoli rabe can be quickly stir-fried. Cook until wilted and the stem parts are tender but not soggy. Cook kale or spinach in a nonstick pan with a little olive oil and garlic, then add a little fresh lemon juice along with a pinch of salt and pepper before serving.

Grilling:
Cut vegetables into chunks and place in a plastic bag. Toss with a small amount of olive oil, chopped garlic, ground pepper, and soy sauce if desired. This is great for sliced mushrooms, zucchini, eggplant, asparagus, bell peppers, and red onions.

Chapter 5: Phase One—Losing Weight

Having cleared out and restocked your pantry, refrigerator, and freezer with green light foods and determined how much weight you want to lose, you are now ready to start Phase One, the weight-loss phase.

We will start logically with breakfast and then work through your day, covering lunch, dinner, and snacks, inserting recipe and meal suggestions as we proceed.

We have included several of the most popular recipes from our earlier books, which have been adapted to meet the important recipe criteria of start-to-table in under thirty minutes.

BREAKFAST

This is the most important meal of the day for three reasons. First, you probably haven't eaten for ten to twelve hours, and the cornerstone of the G.I. Diet is to keep your blood-sugar levels constant and your tummy busy during your waking hours. Second, you will almost certainly overcompensate for a missed breakfast by overeating the rest of the day. Third, a green light breakfast will make you feel light, energetic, well fed, and ready to tackle the day.

For breakfast you have three options, depending on your time availability:

- On the run (10 minutes from start to finish)
- Sit down (10 to 20 minutes)
- Brunch/weekends (20 minutes plus)

ON THE RUN

If time is of the essence, then these are your best bets:

Bran-Delicious Cereal

High-fiber cold cereals (those with 10 grams of fiber or more per serving) with skim milk might not be a lot of fun in themselves, but they can be livened up. Here is a popular blend:

Serves 2
Combine:
1 cup All Bran/High-Fiber Bran
2 cups fresh fruit
1 cup fruit-flavored fat-free yogurt with sweetener
4 tablespoons sliced almonds

Muesli

Virtually all store-bought muesli is a dietary disaster, packed with sugar, fat, and highly processed grains. You can easily make your own green light version in bulk in advance for a yummy fast start to your day.

Makes 3½ cups (about 7 servings)
2 cups old-fashioned rolled oats
¾ cup oat bran
¾ cup sliced almonds
½ cup shelled sunflower seeds
2 tablespoons wheat germ
¼ teaspoon ground cinnamon

1. In a large resealable plastic bag combine all the ingredients. Shake the bag to combine the mixture.

Storage: Keep in a resealable bag or airtight container at room temperature for up to 1 month.

To use: Combine 1/3 cup of muesli with 1/3 cup of milk or water. Cover and refrigerate overnight. In the morning, combine the mixture with one 6-ounce container of nonfat fruit yogurt with sweetener and enjoy cold, or pop it in the microwave for a hot breakfast.

Oatmeal

Oatmeal made with large-flake oats cooked in either water or skim milk for 3 minutes in the microwave is by far my personal favorite, and based on readers' e-mails is the most popular food rediscovery in the G.I. Diet.

Add to either hot or cold cereals one or more of the following:
- fresh/frozen/canned fruit
- nonfat fruit yogurt with sweetener
- sliced almonds/ground flaxseed

Your cereal and topping should be sufficient to fill you, but if not, increase your cereal serving size or add a slice of 100% whole-wheat toast, a pat of light nonhydrogenated margarine and no-sugar-added jam (where fruit is listed as the first ingredient).

Yogurt Fruit Smoothies

While I'm not a big fan of smoothies because the blending process raises the G.I., they can make an occasional quick, healthy change of pace for a fast breakfast.

Serves 2
2 cups skim milk
1 cup nonfat fruit-flavored yogurt with sweetener (or a 6 ounce container)
½ teaspoon sugar substitute
1 cup fresh or frozen berries

1. Combine all the ingredients in a blender and blend until smooth.

TEA/DECAF COFFEE

Normal coffee is out in Phase One, as caffeine increases the appetite. Your best bet is tea or decaf coffee with skim milk, no sugar. If life is completely impossible without your jolt of Java, go for it, but only one cup per day.

SIT DOWN

This is where you have a little extra time to prepare, cook, and eat a broader choice of foods. Most popular choices are usually egg based.

Omelets are easy to make and you can vary them by adding any number of fresh vegetables, a little cheese and/or some meat. You'll find ingredients for a basic omelet here, along with suggestions for making Italian, Mexican, vegetarian, and Western versions. Don't stop with these—using the proportions as a guide, you can add whatever green light ingredients strike your fancy. To round out the meal, include some fresh fruit, a glass of skim milk, or a small carton of nonfat yogurt with sweetener.

Basic Omelet (single serving)

Vegetable oil cooking spray (preferably canola or olive oil)
Additional ingredients (see below)
½ cup liquid egg
¼ cup skim milk

1. Spray the oil in a small nonstick skillet, then place it over a medium heat.

2. Add the mushrooms, bell peppers, broccoli, and/or onion (depending on which omelet you are making), and sauté until tender, about 5 minutes. Transfer the sautéed vegetables to a plate and tent with foil to keep warm.

3. Beat the eggs with the milk and pour them into the skillet. Cook until the eggs start to firm up, then spread the appropriate vegetables, cheese, herbs, beans, and/or meat over them. Continue cooking until the eggs are done to your liking.

Variation: Make scrambled eggs by stirring the eggs as they cook, adding any additional ingredients while the eggs are still soft.

Western

To the basic omelet recipe, add:

2 slices Canadian bacon, lean deli ham, or turkey breast, chopped

1 onion, chopped

1 cup chopped red and green bell peppers

Red pepper flakes

Vegetarian

To the basic omelet recipe, add:

1 ounce grated low-fat cheese

1 cup broccoli florets

½ cup sliced mushrooms

½ cup chopped red and green bell peppers

Italian

To the basic omelet recipe, add:

1 ounce grated nonfat mozzarella cheese

½ cup sliced mushrooms

½ cup tomato purée

Chopped herbs to taste (fresh or dried herbs such as oregano or basil)

Smoked Salmon Scrambled Eggs

This recipe makes scrambled eggs special. Serve with a slice of high-fiber toast.

Serves 2

2 omega-3 eggs plus 3 egg whites

2 tablespoons skim milk

¼ teaspoon black pepper

1 teaspoon canola oil

2 ounces smoked salmon, chopped

1 tablespoon chopped fresh chives or dill

1. Whisk together the eggs, egg whites, milk, and pepper in a medium bowl.

2. Heat the oil in a nonstick skillet over a medium heat. Add the eggs and, using a rubber spatula, gently stir the eggs until almost set. Stir in the salmon and continue to cook, stirring gently, until the eggs are set but still slightly creamy. Stir in the chives.

WEEKEND/BRUNCH

Leisurely brunches are outside the purview of this book. But if you have the time, then you will find some delicious easy recipes in my *Living the G.I. Diet* such as Morning Glory Poached Fruit, Buttermilk Pancakes, and Cinnamon French Toast.

Brunch also gives you a chance to introduce other members of the family or friends to eating the green light way.

LUNCH

For many people, lunch is one meal that is eaten away from home. This poses two challenges. First, what facilities exist for eating out or take-out in your work neighborhood and second, how much time do you have? Let's deal with each in turn.

EATING IN

This usually means taking a bagged lunch to eat at work. You will save time by not having to go out, wait on line to be served, and so on. This also has the advantage of making sure you are completely in control of what you eat. The main downside to this is that you need to set aside time to prepare food at home, though this can be more than offset by the time you will save lunching in at work.

These packed lunches are simple and uncomplicated and require minimal preparation. Most can be done the night before and kept in the refrigerator. They have been grouped into three popular categories of packed lunches: sandwiches, salads, and pasta. I've also added a fast fruit-and-dairy option when you're really pressed for time. The suggestions assume a refrigerator is available at work for food storage.

SANDWICHES

The reason sandwiches are probably the most popular international lunch is they are easy to make, portable, and have endless variation. Here are some guidelines to turn your sandwich into a convenient and filling green-light meal.

- Always use stoneground 100 percent whole-wheat or high-fiber bread
- During Phase One, sandwiches should be eaten open-faced
- Include at least three vegetables, such as lettuce, tomato, red and green bell peppers, cucumber, sprouts, or onion
- Use mustard or hummus as a spread on the bread (no regular mayonnaise or butter)
- Add four ounces of cooked lean meat or fish
- Mix canned tuna or chopped, cooked chicken with low-fat mayonnaise/salad dressing and celery
- Mixed canned salmon with malt vinegar
- To help sandwiches stay fresh, not soggy, pack components separately and assemble them just before eating, if possible

SALADS

Here is a basic salad to which you can add your choice of protein—canned tuna/salmon, sliced cooked chicken breast, lean deli ham, tofu, or even beans.

Basic Salad

Serves 2

3 cups torn or coarsely chopped salad greens, such as romaine, red leaf, mesclun, arugula, or watercress
2 small carrots, grated
1 red, yellow, or green bell pepper, stemmed, seeded, and chopped
2 plum tomatoes, cut into wedges
1 cup sliced cucumber
½ cup chopped red or sweet white onion (Vidalia)

To serve, place the salad greens, carrot, bell pepper, tomato, cucumber, and onion in a bowl and toss to mix. Pour about 1 tablespoon of the basic vinaigrette (see below) over the salad and toss to mix.

Per serving: 1½ cups greens tossed with 1 tablespoon vinaigrette.

Basic Vinaigrette

Makes about ½ cup
2 tablespoons balsamic vinegar
1 teaspoon Dijon mustard
1 teaspoon dried basil
½ teaspoon sugar substitute
½ teaspoon salt
Pinch of freshly ground black pepper
¼ cup extra-virgin olive oil

In a medium bowl, whisk together the vinegar, mustard, basil, sugar substitute, salt, and pepper. Gradually whisk in the oil.

Storage: The vinaigrette will keep in the refrigerator for up to 1 week.

Tip: This vinaigrette is also good tossed with halved cherry tomatoes, cooked green beans, or asparagus.

PASTA

For a great time-saver, cook extra pasta at dinnertime and use it as the basis for a lunch or two. It will keep fresh in the refrigerator for several days. Here is a basic pasta lunch.

Basic Pasta Salad

Serves 1
¾ cup cooked whole-wheat pasta (spirals, shells, or similar shape)
1 cup chopped cooked vegetables (such as broccoli, asparagus, bell peppers, or scallions)
¼ cup light tomato sauce or other low-fat or nonfat pasta sauce
4 ounces chopped cooked chicken or other lean meat, such as ground lean turkey or lean chicken sausage

1. Bring a large pot of water to a boil. Add the pasta and cook until *al dente*, according to the package instructions. Drain the pasta and rinse under cold running water to cool.

2. Place the pasta, vegetables, tomato sauce, and chicken in a bowl and stir to mix well. Refrigerate the salad, covered, until ready to use, then reheat it in the microwave or serve chilled.

Variation: You can use the proportions here as a guide and vary the vegetables, sauce, and source of protein to suit your taste and add variety to your pasta salad lunches.

ON THE RUN

Here is a fast and filling green light option to use occasionally when you are really pushed for time.

Cottage Cheese and Fruit

Serves 1

1 cup low-fat cottage cheese
6 ounces chopped fresh fruit or canned fruit in juice, such as
   peaches, apricots, or pears

Place the cottage cheese and fruit in a plastic bowl with a fitted lid and stir to mix. Store in the refrigerator until lunchtime.

Add half a nutrition bar, such as a Balance or Zone bar, and you're on your way in minutes.

EATING OUT

Sandwiches

If you are under the gun and really don't have time to prepare a bagged lunch, then your best option is a take-out sandwich. Here are some tips on making sure your take-out sandwiches are green light.

- 100% whole-wheat bread
- Hummus or mustard instead of butter, margarine, or mayo
- Slices of chicken/turkey breast, ham, or tuna (avoid mayo, cheese, and bacon bits)

- Lots of vegetables—tomatoes, lettuce, bell peppers, onion rings, sprouts, etc.
- Always remove the top slice of bread and eat your sandwich open-faced

It's a good idea, too, to add a green salad to your sandwich.

FAST FOOD

Another option, if time presses is, believe it or not, a fast-food restaurant. Several of the leading restaurants have introduced menu items that are lower in fat and calories. The main caution is the amount of sodium (salt) that is often added to offset any perceived flavor loss. Another principal villain is the salad dressing, so only use half the packet and avoid creamy dressings. Just beware the minefield of red light temptations!

Here are some green light offerings in some of the major fast-food/take-out food chains.

Note: we strongly recommend that you eat all burgers and sandwiches open-faced, meaning you throw away the top slice of bread or bun. Also only use one third to half of the salad dressing that is normally provided in a packet. They contain far more dressing than you need and add unnecessary calories and salt to your meal.

SUBWAY

Subway is to be congratulated as the pacesetters in the fast-food industry with its broad range of low-fat products. They deserve a G.I. Diet gold star and warrant your support.

6" Sandwiches (all sandwiches included bread, lettuce, tomatoes, onions, green peppers, pickles and olives):
Ham*
Roast Beef*
Turkey Breast*

Turkey Breast and Ham*
Veggie Delite
*High sodium. If blood pressure is a concern, use only fat-free Honey Mustard/Sweet Onion sauces and replace pickles, olives with cucumbers and onions.
Roll: Wheat bread; Honey Oat.

Wraps:
Turkey Breast (high sodium)

Deli-tyle Sandwiches:
Ham
Roast Beef
Turkey Breast

Salads:
Grilled Chicken and Baby Spinach
Subway Club
Veggie Delite

Dressing:
Fat-free Italian

MCDONALD'S
Burgers:
Premium Grilled Chicken Classic (replace the mayo with half a packet of BBQ Sauce)

Salads:
Asian Salad with Grilled Chicken
Bacon Ranch Salad with Grilled Chicken
Caesar Salad with Grilled Chicken
California Cobb Salad with Grilled Chicken
Fruit and Walnut Salad

Dressings:

Newman's Own Low-Fat Balsamic Vinaigrette
Newman's Own Low-Fat Family Recipe Italian
Newman's Own Low-Fat Sesame Ginger

Desserts/Snacks:

Fruit'n'Yogurt Parfait (hold the granola)
Apple dippers with low-fat caramel dip

BURGER KING

Burgers/sandwiches:

Tendergrill Chicken Sandwich with Honey Mustard
Veggie Burger without mayo
Add garden salad to both

Salads:

Tendergrill Chicken Garden Salad
Tendergrill Chicken Caesar Salad

Dressings:

Italian light
Border Ranch

Dessert:

Mott's Strawberry-Flavored Applesauce

WENDY'S

Sandwiches:

Ultimate Chicken Grill Sandwich plus side salad

Salads:

Mandarin Chicken Salad with roasted almonds
Caesar Chicken Salad with roasted almonds

Dressings:
Fat Free French
Reduced Fat Creamy Ranch
Low Fat Honey Mustard

Other:
Large Chili with side salad

TACO BELL
Tacos:
Fresco Style Chicken Ranchero Taco
Fresco Style Taco Supreme

Burritos:
Fresco Style Bean Burrito
Fresco Style Fiesta Burrito—Chicken
Fresco Style Enchirito—Beef
Fresco Style Enchirito—Chicken
Fresco Style Burrito Supreme—Chicken

Gorditas:
Fresco Style Gordita Baja—Chicken
Fresco Style Gordita Supreme—Beef
Fresco Style Gordita Supreme—Chicken

PIZZA HUT
Whereas I recommend avoiding pizza restaurants like the plague, I am delighted to see that Pizza Hut has made a real effort to introduce a line of pizzas and other foods that meet the green light criteria. Let's hope the rest of their competition follows their admirable lead.

Pizzas: (14-inch pizzas—2 slices per serving)
Thin 'N Crispy Pizzas*— Ham, Chicken Supreme or Veggie Lover's
Fit 'N Delicious pizzas—all flavors/combos
*Note: we recommend ordering the Lower Fat Recipe versions of the Thin 'N Crispy Pizzas

Salads:
Garden Salad
Ranch Salad Kits

Dressings:
Lite Ranch
Lite Italian

ARBY'S
Sandwiches:
Hot Ham 'n Cheese
Ham and Swiss Melt

Salads:
Santa Fe with Grilled Chicken
Martha's Vineyard salad

Dressings:
Light Buttermilk Ranch

RESTAURANTS
If you do have the time for a business or working lunch, there are a few simple rules that won't make a lunch any shorter but will help keep you in the green light zone.

Eating out on the G.I. Diet is not difficult today: the trend toward the use of vegetable oils, especially olive oil, more emphasis on broiling/grilling rather than frying, a greater variety of vegetables, increased salad options, and more fish dishes—all make it even easier to dine out the green light way.

As dining out is often a social occasion, you want to be able to enjoy yourself with your friends and not feel that you are putting a damper on the occasion. So here are my top ten suggestions:

1. **Don't go to lunch starving.** Make sure you have a substantial mid-morning snack before you go. This will help reduce the temptation to overeat.

2. Drink water. On arrival, drink a glass of water.

3. Bread Basket. Once the standard basket of rolls or bread has been passed around, which you ignore, ask the waiter to remove whatever is left in the basket, with your co-diners' approval of course. The longer it sits there, the more tempted you will be to dig in.

4. Soup/salad. Order soup or salad first and tell the waiter you would like this as soon as possible. This will stop you from sitting there hungry while others are filling up on the bread. For soups, go for vegetable- or bean-based, the chunkier the better. Avoid cream-based soups. For salads, the golden rule is dressing on the side, as you will only use a fraction of what the restaurant would smother on. And please avoid Caesar salads that come pre-dressed.

5. Double vegetables. As you probably won't get boiled new potatoes and can't be sure what type of rice is being served, ask for a double order of vegetables instead. I have yet to find a restaurant that won't willingly oblige.

6. Meat, poultry, seafood: best options. Stick with low-fat cuts of meat (see shopping guide on page 30) or poultry—if necessary, you can remove the skin. Fish and shellfish are excellent choices but must not be breaded or battered. Remember—as servings tend to be generous in restaurants, eat only 4- to 6-ounce servings (about the size of a pack of cards) and leave the rest.

7. Sauces on side. As with salads, ask for any sauces to be put on the side.

8. Avoid desserts. Desserts are a nutritional minefield, with few green light choices on the whole. Fresh fruit and berries, if available, are your best choice, without the ice cream. Most other choices are a dietary disaster, so my best advice is to try to avoid dessert. If social pressure becomes overwhelming, or it is a special occasion, ask for extra forks so dessert can be shared. A couple of forkfuls with your coffee should get you off the hook with minimal dietary damage!

9. Decaf coffee. Only order decaffeinated coffee. Skim decaf cappuccino is our family's favorite choice.

10. Eat slowly. Finally, and perhaps most importantly, eat slowly. In the eighteenth century, the famous Dr. Johnson reportedly advised chewing food 32 times before swallowing! That's going a little overboard, but at least put your fork down between mouthfuls. The stomach takes 20–30 minutes to let the brain know it feels full. So if you eat quickly, you may be shoveling in more food than you need before the brain says stop. You will also have more time to savor your meal.

DINNER

Typically, we have a little more time available for dinner. The recipes in this section have been designed to take no more than thirty minutes from start to serving time. You can reduce these times even further—see Cooking Basics, page 49, for some additional time saving ideas.

These recipes are simple and easy to prepare and cook and have been devised to feed two.

THE RECIPES

Remember to assemble all ingredients and utensils first. Each recipe is accompanied by suggested sides. If you decide not to include a salad, make sure you add additional vegetables. Check Cooking Basics for preparation instructions. When these sides include rice, potatoes, or pasta, the recipe starts with a reminder so you will bring to the boil the water for these ingredients at the beginning and they will be ready along with the rest of the food.

Tarragon Chicken with Mushrooms

Tarragon adds a light French flavor. The variation below is great for entertaining.

Prep time: **10** minutes Total time: **30** minutes

2 teaspoons vegetable oil
2 chicken cutlets (4 ounces each)
Freshly ground black pepper
1 teaspoon nonhydrogenated margarine
1 small onion, chopped
8 ounces sliced mushrooms
¼ cup vermouth (see note) or white wine

1 teaspoon dried tarragon
½ cup chicken broth (low-fat, low-sodium) or water

Sides Suggestions (see Basics page 50)
1 cup frozen peas
Basmati rice
Salad greens
White-wine vinaigrette

1. Prepare the rice according to the basic instructions. About 2 minutes before the rice is finished cooking, add 1 cup of frozen peas, stir, and simmer for 2 minutes.

2. Meanwhile, heat the oil in a nonstick skillet over a medium-high heat. Sprinkle the chicken with black pepper and sauté until cooked through on both sides (about 6 minutes per side). Remove to a plate and tent with foil while you make the sauce.

3. Melt the margarine in the same pan. Add the onion and mushrooms and sauté until softened, about 5 minutes. Then add the vermouth and tarragon and simmer for 1 minute. Add the broth and simmer for 2 minutes, or until reduced by half. Season with black pepper to taste.

4. Serve the chicken with the rice served alongside and topped with the sauce.

Entertaining Variation: This dish can be made with veal cutlets, and instead of adding peas to the rice you can serve it with steamed green beans or asparagus seasoned with a small amount of lemon juice and black pepper. To prepare the asparagus, see Basics.

Note: Vermouth is a great substitute for white wine and stores well.

Sautéed Chicken Provencal

Prep time: **10** minutes   Total time: **30** minutes

1 tablespoon olive oil
2 chicken cutlets
Freshly ground black pepper
1 clove garlic, finely chopped
½ cup chicken broth (low-fat, low-sodium)
1 teaspoon dried herbes de Provence
½ teaspoon nonhydrogenated margarine
¾ teaspoon lemon juice

Sides Suggestions (see Basics page 50)
4–6 new potatoes
Mixed vegetables
Tomatoes with balsamic vinegar and olive oil

1. Prepare the potatoes following the basic instructions.

2. Meanwhile, heat the oil in a nonstick skillet over a medium-high heat. Sprinkle the chicken with black pepper and sauté until cooked through on both sides (about 6 minutes per side). Remove to a plate and tent with foil to keep warm while you make the sauce.

3. Add the garlic to the same pan and sauté for 1 minute, stirring constantly. Add the broth and herbs and simmer until the broth is reduced by half, about 4 minutes. Stir in the margarine and lemon juice and cook, stirring, for 30 seconds, then serve.

Roasted Chicken with Tomatoes and Asparagus

Prep time: **5** minutes   Total time: **25** minutes

2 cups cherry or grape tomatoes, halved
2 tablespoons olive oil
3 cloves garlic, crushed
1 teaspoon dried tarragon
1 teaspoon hot red pepper flakes, or to taste
2 boneless, skinless chicken breasts
½ teaspoon salt
½ teaspoon black pepper
16 stalks asparagus, trimmed

Sides Suggestions (see Basics page 50)
Basmati rice
Green salad

1. Prepare the rice following the basic instructions and preheat the oven to 450°F.

2. Meanwhile, toss the tomatoes with the olive oil, garlic, tarragon, and red pepper flakes in a large bowl.

3. Place the chicken on a rimmed baking sheet. Pour the tomato mixture over the chicken, arranging the tomatoes in a single layer around the chicken. Sprinkle with the salt and pepper, place in the oven and roast for 20–25 minutes, or until the chicken is no longer pink inside. Transfer the chicken to a serving platter and spoon the tomatoes and juices over the chicken.

4. While the chicken is roasting, steam the asparagus for 3–4 minutes, or until tender-crisp, and prepare the green salad.

Curried Chicken with Snow Peas

Prep time: **5** minutes   Total time: **20** minutes

2 teaspoons olive oil
8 ounces boneless skinless chicken breasts, cubed
1 clove garlic, minced
1 small onion, chopped
2 teaspoons curry powder, or to taste
6 ounces chicken broth (low-fat, low-sodium)
4 ounces low-fat coconut milk
1 carrot, chopped
¼ teaspoon salt
Freshly ground black pepper
2 cups snow peas

Sides Suggestions (see Basics page 50)
Basmati rice
Mixed green salad

1. Prepare the rice following the basic instructions and put up the water for steaming the snow peas.

2. Meanwhile, heat the oil in a nonstick skillet over a medium-high heat. Add the chicken and sauté for about 5 minutes, turning once, until it is no longer pink inside. Remove to a plate and tent with foil to keep warm.

3. Add the garlic, onion, and curry powder to the pan and cook for 2 minutes, or until the onions have softened. Add the broth, coconut milk, carrot, salt, and pepper to taste. Cover and simmer, stirring occasionally, for about 5 minutes, or until the carrot begins to soften. Return the chicken to the skillet and simmer, uncovered, for about 5 minutes.

4. Meanwhile, steam the snow peas for 2–3 minutes (or 1 minute in the microwave). Gently stir the snow peas into the rice and top with the chicken mixture. Serve with the salad.

Chicken Stir-Fry

You can use your favorite variation of vegetables for this dish.

Prep time: **10** minutes   Total time: **25** minutes

1 teaspoon sesame oil
8 ounces boneless, skinless chicken breasts, chopped
1 cup sliced mushrooms
1 small onion, chopped
1 clove garlic, finely chopped
2 teaspoons grated fresh ginger
1 red bell pepper, stemmed, seeded, and chopped
1 carrot, chopped
1 stalk celery, chopped
1 tablespoon soy sauce
1 cup bean sprouts

Sides Suggestions (see Basics page 50)
Basmati rice prepared with chicken broth
Romaine lettuce salad

1. Cook the rice following the basic instructions and prepare the salad.

2. Heat the oil in a large nonstick skillet over a medium-high heat. Add the chicken, mushrooms, onion, garlic, and ginger and sauté for about 8 minutes, or until the chicken is no longer pink inside. Add the bell pepper, carrot, celery, and soy sauce. Cook, stirring, for 2 minutes. Add the bean sprouts and toss to combine.

3. Serve the chicken with the rice and salad alongside.

Chicken Peperonata

| ⏱ Prep time: **10** minutes | ⏱ Total time: **30** minutes |

2 boneless, skinless chicken breasts
1 tablespoon whole-wheat flour
2 teaspoons olive oil
1 small onion, sliced
1 clove garlic, minced
1 red bell pepper, stemmed, seeded, and thinly sliced
½ yellow or green bell pepper, stemmed, seeded, and thinly
  sliced
1 can (14-ounce) chopped tomatoes
¼ cup sun-dried tomatoes, chopped
½ teaspoon dried oregano
¼ teaspoon salt
¼ teaspoon black pepper

Sides Suggestions (see Basics page 50)
Pasta or rice
Mixed salad

1. Prepare the pasta or rice following the basic instructions.

2. Coat the chicken breasts with the flour. Heat the oil in a large nonstick skillet over a medium-high heat. Add the chicken and brown on both sides. Remove to a plate and tent with foil while you prepare the vegetables.

3. Add the onion and garlic to the skillet and cook until softened, about 5 minutes. Add the bell peppers, chopped tomatoes, sun-dried tomatoes, oregano, salt, and pepper and bring to a boil. Place the chicken on top of the mixture, then reduce the heat and cook, covered, for 15–20 minutes, or until the chicken is no longer pink inside.

4. Serve the chicken with the pasta or rice and salad.

Sautéed Chicken with Indian Rice

2 teaspoons canola oil
2 boneless, skinless chicken breasts
Freshly ground black pepper
1 small onion, chopped
1 clove garlic, chopped
2 teaspoons garam masala
½ cup basmati rice
12 ounces chicken broth (low-fat, low-sodium)

Sides Suggestions (see Basics page 50)
Baby bok choy or Asian vegetable mix

1. Heat 1 teaspoon of the oil in a nonstick skillet over a medium-high heat. Sprinkle the chicken with black pepper, add it to the skillet, and cook for about 6 minutes on each side, or until no longer pink inside. Remove to a plate and tent with foil to keep warm while you make the rice.

2. Heat the remaining teaspoon of oil in a medium saucepan over a medium heat, and add the onion and garlic. Sauté until the onion has softened, about 5 minutes. Stir in the garam masala and cook for 30 seconds. Add the rice, stir and cook for 3 minutes, stirring to coat the rice in the oil.

3. Stir in the broth, bring to a boil, then reduce the heat and simmer, covered, for 10–12 minutes, or until the rice is done.

4. Serve the chicken with the rice and baby bok choy alongside.

Hint: This rice is also great with fish. For a vegetarian version of the rice, use vegetable broth instead of chicken broth.

Chicken Fingers with Apricot-Mustard Dipping Sauce

⏱ Prep time: **5** minutes	⏱ Total time: **15** minutes

(plus marinating overnight)

1 egg white
1 tablespoon soy sauce
1 small clove garlic, minced
8 ounces boneless, skinless chicken breasts, cut into ½-inch strips
½ cup toasted sesame seeds (see note)
1 teaspoon canola oil
For the dipping sauce
3 tablespoons high-fruit apricot preserves
¼ cup water
1 tablespoon Dijon mustard

Sides Suggestions (see Basics page 50)
Grilled zucchini and eggplant slices
A plate of cut-up raw vegetables

1. Preheat the oven to 375°F. Whisk together the egg white, soy sauce, and garlic in a large bowl. Add the chicken and toss to coat. Cover and refrigerate for at least 1 hour and up to 1 day.

2. Remove the chicken from the marinade, allowing the excess to drip off. Sprinkle all sides of the chicken with sesame seeds and place on a baking sheet brushed with oil. Bake for 5 minutes on each side, or until the chicken is no longer pink inside.

3. While the chicken is baking, make the dipping sauce by whisking together all the ingredients in a small bowl.

4. Serve the chicken with the dipping sauce along with the zucchini, eggplant, and raw vegetables.

Note: To toast the sesame seeds, roast them in a preheated 300°F oven for 10 minutes, stirring a couple of times. Make extra and store them in an airtight jar in the refrigerator.

Super-Express Oriental Salmon with Leeks

So easy and delicious. If you're using frozen fish, increase the cooking time by a couple of minutes.

Prep time: 5 minutes	Total time: **15** minutes

1 tablespoon soy sauce
1 tablespoon lemon juice
½ teaspoon ground ginger
Freshly ground black pepper
1 leek, thinly sliced (white and light-green part only)
2 salmon fillets (4–5 ounces each)

Sides Suggestions (see Basics page 50)
Basmati rice
Wilted greens

1. Prepare the rice following the basic instructions.

2. Meanwhile, combine the soy sauce, lemon juice, ginger, and black pepper to taste in a microwaveable dish. Add the leek, then the fish, turning once to coat.

3. Cover the dish with plastic wrap, leaving a small gap for steam to be released. Microwave on high for about 5 minutes, or until the fish is opaque and flakes easily with a fork. If your microwave does not rotate, turn the dish after 2½ minutes.

4. Serve the fish along with the rice and greens.

Tomato and Cheese Catfish

An easy weeknight dish.

Prep time: **5** minutes   Total time: **25** minutes

1 medium tomato, chopped
2 green onions, chopped
1 small clove garlic, minced
½ small chili, seeded and minced
1 tablespoon lemon juice
2 teaspoons grated lemon zest
1 teaspoon olive oil
¼ teaspoon salt
¼ teaspoon black pepper
2 catfish or tilapia fillets (4 ounces each)
3 tablespoons low-fat cheddar cheese

Sides Suggestions (see Basics page 50)
Whole-wheat pasta
Green beans
Tossed salad

1. Prepare the pasta following the basic instructions and preheat the oven to 425°F.

2. Meanwhile, toss together the tomato, onion, garlic, chili, lemon juice, lemon zest, olive oil, salt, and pepper in a medium bowl.

3. Arrange the catfish fillets in a small baking dish; top with the tomato mixture and sprinkle with the cheese. Bake for 15–20 minutes, or until the fish flakes easily with a fork.

4. Serve the fish with the pasta, green beans, and salad.

Stir-Fried Scallops in Black Bean Sauce

Prep time: **15** minutes   Total time: **25** minutes

½ cup chicken or fish broth (low-fat, low-sodium) or water
1 teaspoon cornstarch
1 tablespoon black bean sauce
1 clove garlic, minced
1 teaspoon sesame oil
2 teaspoons canola oil
1 stalk celery, chopped
½ red bell pepper, stemmed, seeded, and chopped
3 ounces shiitake mushrooms, stemmed and sliced
1 cup shredded green cabbage
7–8 raw scallops
2 green onions, sliced on the diagonal
2 tablespoons chopped fresh cilantro (optional)

Sides Suggestions (see Basics page 50)
Basmati rice
Salad

1. Prepare the rice following the basic instructions.

2. Whisk together the broth, cornstarch, black bean sauce, garlic and sesame oil in a small bowl.

3. Heat the canola oil in a wok or large nonstick skillet over a medium-high heat. Add the celery, red pepper, mushrooms, and cabbage and stir-fry for about 5 minutes, or until the cabbage is tender-crisp.

4. Add the scallops, green onions, and sauce. Stir-fry until the scallops are cooked and the sauce is thickened, about 3 minutes. Garnish with the cilantro, if using.

5. Serve the scallops with the rice and salad.

Braised Whitefish

You can also use haddock, tilapia, or catfish in this dish.

| Prep time: 5 minutes | Total time: 25 minutes |

2 Pacific halibut steaks (4 ounces each)
2 teaspoons grainy mustard
2 teaspoons lemon zest
1/4 teaspoon black pepper
1 teaspoon olive oil
1/2 onion, chopped
4 cloves garlic, peeled
Large handful of fresh spinach
1/8 teaspoon salt
1/2 cup vermouth or dry white wine

Sides Suggestions (see Basics page 50)
New potatoes
Stir-fried lemony vegetables

1. Prepare the potatoes following the basic instructions. Preheat the oven to 400°F.

2. Rinse the fish and pat dry with paper towels. Stir together the mustard, lemon zest, and pepper in a small bowl. Coat the fish on all sides with the mixture and set aside.

3. Heat the oil in a large ovenproof skillet over a medium-high heat. Add the onion and garlic and cook for 5 minutes, or until softened. Reduce the heat to medium and stir in the spinach and salt. Add the vermouth or wine. Place the fish on top of the spinach mixture; cover and bake for 15 minutes, or until the fish flakes with a fork.

4. Serve the fish with the new potatoes and vegetables.

Sautéed Halibut with Tomatoes and Anchovies

Halibut is a delicious firm fish. Double the recipe and you have a dish suitable for dinner guests.

🕐 Prep time: **5** minutes	🕐 Total Time: **20** minutes

1 tablespoon olive oil
2 halibut fillets (about 4 ounces each)
Pinch of salt
Freshly ground black pepper
2 cloves garlic, minced
1/8 teaspoon hot pepper flakes, or to taste
4 anchovies, chopped
2 tablespoons chopped flat-leaf parsley
3 plum tomatoes, chopped and seeded

Sides Suggestions (see Basics page 50)
Linguine
Asparagus
Mixed green salad

1. Prepare the pasta following the basic instructions.

2. Heat half the oil in a nonstick skillet over a medium-high heat. Season the fish with the salt and pepper. Sauté for 1 minute on each side, then cover, reduce the heat to medium-low, and cook for 5 minutes, or until the fish is cooked through.

3. Remove the fish to a plate and tent with foil to keep warm. Add the remaining oil to the pan and increase the heat to medium. Add the garlic, pepper flakes, anchovies, and parsley and cook for 3 minutes. Add the tomatoes and cook for 2 minutes.

4. Serve the sauce over the fish with the linguine, asparagus, and salad.

Citrus Fish Steaks

In South American cuisine, fish is "cooked" in citrus juices, sitting for at least six hours. Here we provide a tangy citrus flavor the express way.

🕐 Prep time: **5** minutes	🕐 Total time: **20** minutes

(includes 10 minutes marinating)

2 marlin, shark, or tuna steaks (4 ounces each)
For the marinade
1 tablespoon olive oil
½ teaspoon dried thyme
1 clove garlic, minced
1 teaspoon lemon juice
1 teaspoon lime juice
¼ teaspoon black pepper

Sides Suggestions (see Basics page 50)
Basmati rice
Green beans or fennel

1. Prepare the rice according to the basic instructions.

2. Make the marinade by whisking together all the ingredients in a medium bowl. Place the fish steaks in a small dish and pour over the marinade. Turn to coat and let sit for 10 minutes.

3. Heat a grill or a nonstick pan over a medium-high heat. Remove the fish from the marinade and cook for about 4 minutes on each side, until medium-rare or until desired doneness.

4. Serve the fish with the rice and green beans.

Coconut Curry Shrimp

Don't be alarmed by the long ingredients list—this dish takes just minutes to assemble.

Prep time: **10** minutes   Total time: **20** minutes

2 tablespoons orange juice
1 tablespoon fish sauce
   (optional)
1 teaspoon cornstarch
2 teaspoons soy sauce
1 teaspoon canola oil
8 large shrimps
1 small onion, chopped
1 clove garlic, minced
½ teaspoon green curry
   powder (or to taste)
1 red bell pepper, stemmed,
   seeded, and sliced

¼ cup light coconut milk
1 tablespoon lime juice
1 teaspoon sugar substitute
¼ cup chopped cilantro
1 tablespoon chopped
   unsalted peanuts

*Sides Suggestions (see Basics
   page 50)*
Basmati rice or spaghetti
Sugar-snap peas
Spinach, arugula, and
   watercress salad

1. Prepare the rice or pasta following the basic instructions.

2. Whisk together the orange juice, fish sauce, if using, cornstarch, soy sauce, and canola oil in a medium bowl. Stir in the shrimp and marinate for 5 minutes.

3. Heat the oil in a large nonstick skillet over a medium-high heat. Add the onion and garlic and sauté for 5 minutes, or until softened. Add the curry powder and cook for 1 minute. Add the red peppers and shrimp and cook for 2–3 minutes, or until the shrimp turn pink. Stir in the coconut milk, lime juice, and sugar substitute and cook for 2 minutes.

4. Garnish with the cilantro and peanuts and serve with the rice, peas, and salad.

Note: If you'd like to use cooked shrimp, then add them during the last 30 seconds of cooking time just to warm through.

Salmon, Red Potato, and Asparagus Salad

Prep time: **5–10** minutes   Total time: **15** minutes

8 ounces asparagus, tough ends removed and cut diagonally
  into 1-inch pieces
4 cups salad greens or baby spinach
6 ounces cooked salmon or 1 can (4-ounce) salmon
6 new red potatoes, boiled and quartered
1 cup grape or cherry tomatoes, cut in half
3 green onions, chopped
2 tablespoons chopped fresh mint
For the vinaigrette
2 tablespoons extra-virgin olive oil
2 tablespoons lemon juice
½ teaspoon grated lemon zest (optional)
¼ teaspoon salt
¼ teaspoon black pepper

1. In a steamer basket placed over a pot of boiling water,
steam the asparagus, covered, until tender-crisp, about 5
minutes. Rinse the asparagus under cold running water until
cool, then set aside.

2. To make the vinaigrette: Whisk together the olive oil, lemon
juice, lemon zest, if using, salt, and pepper in a small bowl.

3. Toss the salad greens with half the vinaigrette and divide
between two plates. Break the salmon into bite-size chunks
and place in a large bowl. If using canned salmon, drain, place
in a bowl, and mash lightly. Add the potatoes, asparagus,
tomatoes, green onions, and mint, and carefully toss with the
remaining dressing. Spoon over the greens.

Express Cocoa Spice-Rubbed Grilled Steak

Prep time: 5 minutes   Total time: **15** minutes
to make the rub

2 tablespoons Cocoa Spice Rub (see page 89)
1 tablespoon olive oil
1 clove garlic, minced
2 top sirloin grilling steaks (4 ounces each)

Sides Suggestions (see Basics page 50)
New potatoes or rice
Green salad
Sugar-snap peas
Grilled portobello mushrooms or other vegetables

1. Cook the potatoes or rice following the basic instructions.

2. Combine the rub mix, olive oil, and garlic in a small bowl. Rub the mixture into all sides of the steak. Place the steak on a greased grill over a medium-high heat and grill for about 8 minutes, turning once, until medium-rare. Grill the mushrooms at the same time.

3. Slice the steak thinly and serve on top of a green salad along with the potatoes, peas, and mushrooms.

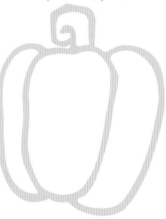

Cocoa Spice Rub

Makes approximately ⅓ cup
2 tablespoons cocoa powder
2 teaspoons ground turmeric
1 teaspoon ground cumin
1 teaspoon ground coriander
1 teaspoon ground allspice
1 teaspoon ground cardamom
½ teaspoon salt
½ teaspoon black pepper

1. Mix all the ingredients together in a small bowl. Store in an airtight container for up to 6 months.

Beef and Bowties

(⏱) Prep time: **5** minutes	(◑) Total time: **25** minutes

3 ounces whole-wheat bowtie pasta
6 ounces extra-lean ground beef
1 small onion, chopped
2 cloves garlic, minced
½ zucchini, chopped
½ red bell pepper, stemmed, seeded, and chopped
4 ounces mushrooms, chopped
2 medium tomatoes, chopped
½ cup tomato sauce
2 teaspoons dried basil
¼ teaspoon salt
½ teaspoon black pepper
2 tablespoons chopped fresh flat-leaf parsley

Sides Suggestions (see Basics page 50)
Light Caesar salad

1. Bring a large pot of water to a boil, add the pasta, and cook until *al dente*, about 10 minutes. Drain.

2. Combine the beef and onion in a large nonstick skillet over a medium-high heat. Cook until the beef is browned, stirring constantly, about 8 minutes. Add the garlic, zucchini, red pepper, and mushrooms and cook, stirring occasionally, until the vegetables have softened, about 6 minutes.

3. Add the tomatoes, tomato sauce, basil, salt, and pepper, and simmer for 5 minutes. Stir in the pasta and parsley and serve along with the salad.

Vegetarian option: Use vegetarian ground beef (such as a crumbled Boca burger), adding it after the onion has softened.

Chili con Carne

Always a favorite, this quick version still has great flavor. You can double the recipe and freeze half for another day.

| Prep time: **10** minutes | Total time: **30** minutes |

8 ounces extra-lean ground beef
1 onion, chopped
1 red bell pepper, stemmed, seeded, and chopped
1 green bell pepper, stemmed, seeded, and chopped
1 can (28-ounce) chopped tomatoes
1 cup water
1 tablespoon chili powder, or to taste
½ teaspoon ground cumin (optional)
1 teaspoon dried basil
1 teaspoon dried oregano
1 can (19-ounce) red kidney beans, drained and rinsed
1 cup corn niblets
2 tablespoon nonfat or low-fat sour cream or 2 teaspoons low-fat shredded cheddar cheese

Sides Suggestions (see Basics page 50)
Mixed green salad

1. Combine the beef and onions in a deep nonstick skillet over a medium-high heat. Cook until the beef is browned, stirring constantly, about 8 minutes. Add the bell peppers, tomatoes, water, chili powder, cumin (if using), basil, and oregano. Bring to a boil, then lower the heat, cover, and simmer for 20 minutes.

2. Add the beans and corn niblets and cook for 2 minutes. Serve with a dollop of sour cream along with the salad.

Vegetarian options: Use vegetarian ground beef (such as a crumbled Boca burger) or ½ cup of bulgur, adding it after the onion has softened.

Hint: You can vary the vegetables according to your taste.

Pork Tenderloin with Apple and Rosemary

Prep time: **5** minutes   Total time: **30** minutes

2 teaspoons canola oil
8 ounces pork tenderloin, cut into 2 pieces
1 small onion, thinly sliced
½ teaspoon dried rosemary or 1 teaspoon chopped fresh
   rosemary
¼ teaspoon curry powder (optional)
¼ cup apple juice
1 teaspoon cider vinegar
1 firm apple, cored, halved, and thinly sliced
2 teaspoons currants

Sides Suggestions (see Basics page 50)
Basmati rice or new potatoes
Brussels sprouts

1. Prepare the rice or potatoes following the basic instructions.

2. Meanwhile, heat the oil in a nonstick skillet over a medium-high heat. Sear the pork on all sides, then remove to a plate and tent with foil.

3. Lower the heat to medium-low, add the onion, rosemary, and curry powder, if using, and cook until the onions soften, about 5 minutes. Add the apple juice and vinegar and cook for 2 minutes. Add the apples and currants and return the pork to the pan. Cover and cook for about 15 minutes, until the pork is just cooked through.

4. Slice the pork and serve with the apples and onions, with the rice or potatoes and Brussels sprouts alongside.

Speedy Pork and Lentils

Prep time: **15** minutes   Total time: **30** minutes

½ cup lentils
1½ cups water
1 small lemon wedge
½ celeriac, peeled and cut into ½-inch chunks
2 teaspoons olive oil
¼ teaspoon dried thyme
Pinch of salt
Pinch of black pepper
1 small onion, chopped
1 small clove garlic, minced
6 ounces pork tenderloin, sliced
¼ cup dry Marsala or red wine
1 teaspoon Dijon mustard

Sides Suggestions (see Basics page 50)
Mixed green salad
Sliced tomatoes with balsamic vinaigrette

1. Preheat the oven to 425°F.

2. Place the lentils, water, and lemon in a medium pot over a high heat. Bring to a boil, then reduce the heat and simmer for 20 minutes, or until the lentils are tender. Drain and return the lentils to the pot, discarding the lemon wedge.

3. Meanwhile, place the celeriac on a rimmed baking sheet and toss with 1 teaspoon of the olive oil, the thyme, salt, and pepper. Roast for 15 minutes, or until the celeriac is just tender. Add to the pot with the lentils.

4. Heat the remaining teaspoon of oil in a nonstick skillet over a medium-high heat. Add the onion and garlic and cook for 5 minutes, or until softened. Add the pork and cook for 2–3 minutes, or until the pork is browned but still slightly pink inside. Stir in the Marsala and mustard and bring to a boil. Reduce the heat slightly and cook for 2 minutes, or until the sauce is slightly thickened.

5. Serve the pork over the lentils and celeriac, along with the salad and tomatoes.

Pork Chops with Pear and Ginger

Apples may be substituted for the pears.

Prep time: **10** minutes   Total time: **25** minutes

2 boneless pork loin chops, trimmed of fat
¼ teaspoon salt
¼ teaspoon black pepper
1 teaspoon olive oil
1 leek (white and light-green parts only), halved lengthwise and
   sliced
1 Bosc pear, cored and cut into eighths
2 teaspoons minced fresh ginger
½ teaspoon sugar substitute
½ cup chicken broth (low-sodium, low-fat)
1 tablespoon apple-cider vinegar

Sides Suggestions (see Basics page 50)
Rice to soak up the sauce
Sautéed spinach or kale

1. Prepare the rice following the basic instructions.

2. Meanwhile, sprinkle the pork chops on both sides with salt and pepper. Heat the oil in a nonstick skillet over a medium-high heat. Add the pork chops and cook for 3–4 minutes per side, or until just a slight hint of pink remains in the center. Remove to a plate and tent with foil.

3. Add the leek, pear, and ginger to the skillet, then sprinkle with the sugar substitute. Cook, stirring frequently, until the leeks are softened and the pears are beginning to turn golden. Pour in the chicken broth and apple-cider vinegar and simmer for 3–5 minutes, or until the pears are softened and the sauce is reduced slightly. Return the pork and any accumulated juices to the skillet. Simmer for 2 minutes, or until the pork is heated through.

4. Serve the pork with the rice and spinach or kale.

Veal Piccata

Prep time: **5** minutes   Total time: **25** minutes

8 ounces veal cutlets
½ teaspoon salt
¼ teaspoon black pepper
2 teaspoons extra-virgin olive oil
8 ounces mushrooms, sliced
1 can (14-ounce) artichoke hearts, drained and halved
1 teaspoon dried sage leaves
2 tablespoons lemon juice
½ teaspoon lemon zest
2 tablespoons chopped fresh flat-leaf parsley

Sides Suggestions (see Basics page 50)
New potatoes
Green beans

1. Prepare the potatoes following the basic instructions.

2. Sprinkle the veal cutlets with ¼ teaspoon of the salt and the pepper.

3. Heat 1 teaspoon of the oil in a large nonstick skillet over a medium-high heat. Add the veal and sear for 2 minutes on each side, or until browned with just a slight hint of pink remaining. Remove to a plate and tent with foil to keep warm.

4. Return the skillet to the heat and add the remaining teaspoon of oil. Add the mushrooms, artichokes, sage, and remaining ¼ teaspoon of salt and cook for 15 minutes, or until the mushrooms have released their liquid and are beginning to brown. Add the lemon juice and zest and simmer for 1 minute.

5. Pour the sauce over the veal and sprinkle with the parsley. Serve with the potatoes and green beans.

Express Sautéed Greens with Ginger

| Prep time: **5** minutes | Total time: **15** minutes |

2 teaspoons canola oil
1 small onion, chopped
4 baby bok choy, chopped coarsely
4 cups chopped kale (tough stem ends removed)
1/4 cup vegetable broth (low-fat, low-sodium) or water
2 tablespoons soy sauce
1/2 teaspoon toasted sesame oil (optional)
1 clove garlic, finely chopped
1 tablespoon finely chopped fresh ginger
1 1/2 cups canned chickpeas or other beans, drained and rinsed
1 tablespoon sesame seeds, toasted (optional)

Sides Suggestions (see Basics page 50)
Top with cooked chicken or turkey breast slices or add 4 ounces
   cubed tofu with the garlic and ginger

1. Heat the oil in a nonstick skillet or wok over a medium-high heat. Add the onion and sauté until softened, about 3 minutes. Add the bok choy and kale and sauté for 2 minutes, or until slightly softened. Add the broth, soy sauce, and sesame oil, if using, and bring to a boil. Add the garlic and ginger. Reduce the heat to medium, cover the skillet, and cook for 5 minutes, or until the vegetables are tender-crisp.

2. Add the chickpeas and simmer until they are warmed through. Sprinkle with the sesame seeds, if using, and serve with the chicken.

Curried Quinoa Salad

Adjust the amount of curry powder to give this salad more or less of a kick.

🕐 Prep time: **20** minutes	🌙 Total time: **30** minutes

Serves 2–3

½ cup quinoa, rinsed and drained
Pinch of salt (1)
1 tablespoon plus 2 teaspoons olive oil
2 teaspoons chopped shallot
½ teaspoon curry powder, or to taste
1 tablespoon lemon juice
½ teaspoon Dijon mustard
Pinch of salt (2)
Pinch of black pepper

1 small carrot, finely chopped
¼ red bell pepper, stemmed, seeded, and finely chopped
4 dried apricots, chopped
3–4 cashews, chopped
1 green onion, chopped
2 teaspoons chopped flat-leaf parsley

Sides Suggestions (see Basics page 50)
Soy chicken strips
Broccoli spears

1. Place a nonstick skillet over a medium heat. Add the quinoa and pan-roast for 5 minutes, or until fragrant and beginning to pop. In a small saucepan, bring 1 cup of water to a boil over a high heat. Add the roasted quinoa and a pinch of salt; cover, reduce the heat, and simmer for 15 minutes, or until the water has been absorbed. Transfer the quinoa to a large bowl and set aside to cool.

2. Now heat 1 tablespoon of the olive oil in the same skillet over a medium-high heat. Add the shallot and sauté for 3 minutes, or until softened. Stir in the curry powder and cook, stirring, for another 2 minutes. Remove from the heat and set aside.

3. Whisk together the remaining 2 teaspoons of olive oil, the lemon juice, mustard, salt, and pepper in a small bowl and pour the mixture over the quinoa. Stir in the carrot, bell pepper, apricots, cashews, green onion, and parsley. This dish can be covered and refrigerated for up to 3 days.

Non-vegetarian option: Add a few slices of grilled chicken.

Creamy Garlic Fettuccine with Tofu and Broccoli Rabe

A low-G.I. cream sauce! You can also use Swiss chard, broccoli, or chopped asparagus in place of the broccoli rabe.

Prep time: **10** minutes		Total time: **25** minutes	

½ cup low-fat cottage cheese
2 tablespoons light cream cheese
1 tablespoon grated Parmesan cheese
1 small clove garlic, minced
⅛ teaspoon ground nutmeg
⅛ teaspoon black pepper
2 teaspoons olive oil
1 cup cubed firm tofu
3 ounces whole-wheat fettuccine or linguine
½ bunch broccoli rabe, chopped

Sides Suggestions (see Basics page 50)
Romaine lettuce salad

1. Combine the cottage cheese, cream cheese, Parmesan, garlic, nutmeg and pepper in a food processor and process until smooth.

2. Heat the oil in a nonstick skillet over a medium-high heat. Add the tofu and brown on all sides, about 2 minutes, then remove to a plate.

3. Bring a large pot of salted water to a boil. Add the fettuccine and cook for 6 minutes. Add the broccoli rabe and cook for 3–4 minutes, or until the fettuccine is *al dente* and the broccoli rabe is tender-crisp. Drain well and return to the pot, then add the tofu and the cheese mixture, tossing to coat well with the sauce.

4. Serve along with the salad.

Eggplant Parmesan

Prep time: **5** minutes   Total time: **20–25** minutes

1 tablespoon grated Parmesan cheese
1 teaspoon Italian herb seasoning
¼ teaspoon salt
¼ teaspoon black pepper
1 medium eggplant, cut into ½-inch slices
1 tablespoon olive oil
½ cup pasta sauce, heated
2 tablespoons shredded part-skim mozzarella cheese
1 tablespoon chopped fresh Italian parsley or basil (optional)

Sides Suggestions (see Basics page 50)
Meat-alternative sausages, burgers, or steaks or cooked turkey
   breast slices or extra-lean cooked beef slices
Whole-wheat noodles
Roasted tomatoes and peas
Mixed salad

1. Prepare the pasta following the basic instructions.

2. Combine the Parmesan cheese, Italian herb seasoning, salt, and pepper in a small bowl. Brush the eggplant slices with oil and sprinkle the herb mixture on both sides of the slices.

3. Place the eggplant on a greased grill over a medium-high heat. Close the lid and grill for about 15–20 minutes, turning once, until tender. Place the eggplant in a shallow dish. Pour the pasta sauce over the top and sprinkle with the mozzarella and parsley, if using. Serve with the meat alternative, noodles, and vegetables.

Skillet option: If a grill is unavailable you can cook the eggplant in a nonstick skillet or grill pan with 2 teaspoons of olive oil.

Moroccan-Spiced Vegetable Ragout

Don't let the long ingredients list deter you—this richly flavored dish is still quick to prepare and makes a complete meal served over basmati rice.

> Prep time: **15** minutes   Total time: **30–35** minutes

1½ teaspoons olive oil
½ pound eggplant, cut into 1-inch pieces
1 small onion, sliced
2 small cloves garlic, minced
1 teaspoon minced fresh ginger
1 teaspoon garam masala
1½ teaspoons tomato paste
1½ cups vegetable broth
1 cup cauliflower florets
1 carrot, cut into 1-inch pieces
½ red bell pepper, stemmed, seeded, and chopped
½ can (14-ounce) chickpeas, drained and rinsed
¼ cup dried apricots, sliced
2 tablespoons raisins
¼ teaspoon salt
¼ teaspoon black pepper
¼ cup black olives, pitted (optional)
2 tablespoons chopped fresh cilantro

Sides Suggestions (see Basics page 50)
Basmati rice
Salad

1. Prepare the rice following the basic instructions.

2. Heat the oil in a large saucepan or Dutch oven over a medium-high heat. Add the eggplant, onion, garlic, ginger, and garam masala and cook for 8 minutes, or until the vegetables have softened. Stir in the tomato paste.

3. Add the broth, cauliflower, carrot, bell pepper, chickpeas, apricots, raisins, salt, and pepper. Cover and simmer for 15–20 minutes, or until the vegetables are tender. Stir in the olives, if using, and the cilantro and serve with the rice and salad.

Quick Tofu with Penne and Feta

Prep time: 5 minutes	Total time: **15–20** minutes

3 ounces whole-wheat penne
2 teaspoons olive oil
7 ounces extra-firm herbed tofu cut into ½-inch cubes (see note)
1 small clove garlic, finely chopped
½ zucchini, chopped
½ green bell pepper, stemmed, seeded, and chopped
½ teaspoon dried oregano
½ teaspoon dried basil
Pinch of salt
Pinch of black pepper
2 large tomatoes, seeded and chopped
2 tablespoons balsamic vinegar
4 ounces reduced-fat feta cheese, crumbled

1. Bring a large pot of water to a boil. Add the pasta and cook until *al dente*, according to the package instructions. Drain.

2. Meanwhile, heat 1 teaspoon of the oil in a nonstick skillet over a medium-high heat. Add the tofu and brown on all sides, about 2 minutes. Add the garlic, zucchini, bell pepper, oregano, basil, salt, and pepper and cook for 2–3 minutes, until the vegetables have started to soften. Add the tomatoes and vinegar and cook for another 2–3 minutes, until the tomato has softened.

3. Add the pasta to the skillet, then add the cheese and stir gently.

Note: If herbed tofu is not available, use plain and increase the amount of dried herbs.

Use these salads with cooked poultry breast, lean deli meats, fish and seafood, or meat alternatives for a quick dinner. They all make great side dishes.

Mixed Bean Salad

Prep time: **10** minutes   Total time: **15** minutes

Serves 2–3
8 ounces green beans, trimmed and cut into 1-inch pieces
1 can mixed beans (14-ounce), drained and rinsed
1 red bell pepper, stemmed, seeded, and chopped
¼ cup chopped red onion
2 tablespoons red-wine vinegar
1 tablespoon extra-virgin olive oil
1 clove garlic, minced
1 teaspoon Dijon mustard
Pinch of salt
Pinch of black pepper
1 tablespoon chopped fresh flat-leaf parsley
2 cups shredded romaine lettuce

1. Bring a medium saucepan of water to a boil. Add the green beans and cook for 5 minutes, or microwave on high for 3 minutes, or until tender-crisp. Drain and rinse under cold running water until cool, then drain well again.

2. Place the green beans in a large bowl. Add the mixed beans, red pepper, and red onion.

3. Whisk together the vinegar, oil, garlic, mustard, salt, and pepper in a small bowl. Pour the dressing over the bean mixture. Add the parsley and toss to coat evenly.

4. Divide the lettuce between 2 or 3 plates. Spoon the bean mixture over the lettuce and serve.

Warm Spinach and Bacon Salad with Cranberry Vinaigrette

This bistro-style salad makes a satisfying lunch.

Prep time: **10** minutes   Total time: **15** minutes

4 slices Canadian bacon
5 ounces fresh baby spinach
1 small apple, chopped
$\frac{1}{4}$ cup cranberry juice
2 teaspoons red-wine vinegar
1 teaspoon Dijon mustard
$\frac{1}{4}$ teaspoon sugar substitute
Pinch of salt
Pinch of black pepper
2 teaspoons dried cranberries
1 tablespoon roasted sunflower seeds

1. Cook the bacon in a nonstick skillet over a medium-high heat until crisp, about 5 minutes. Remove from the pan and drain on paper towels. Let the bacon cool and chop into small pieces.

2. Toss together the spinach and apple in a large bowl.

3. Whisk together the cranberry juice, vinegar, mustard, sugar substitute, salt, and pepper in a small saucepan. Add the cranberries and place the saucepan over a medium heat. Heat the dressing until just warmed.

4. Pour the dressing over the salad and toss to coat. Sprinkle with the bacon and sunflower seeds and toss again. Serve immediately.

Super Express: Cold Noodle Salad with Cucumbers and Sesame Seeds

Fancy enough for guests but takes only minutes to make.

Prep time: **5** minutes   Total time: **10** minutes

3 ounces thin whole-wheat noodles
4 teaspoons rice vinegar
1 teaspoon sugar substitute
2 teaspoons soy sauce
1 tablespoon toasted sesame seeds
¼ cucumber, seeded, quartered, and sliced
¼ cup grated carrot
1 green onion, sliced on diagonal

Sides Suggestions (see Basics page 50)
Cooked fish or chicken
Asian vegetable mix

1. Bring a large pot of water to a boil. Add the noodles and cook until *al dente*, according to the package instructions. Drain and rinse under cold running water, then transfer to a large bowl.

2. Whisk together the vinegar, sugar substitute, and soy sauce in a small bowl. Pour the dressing over the noodles and stir in the sesame seeds, cucumber, carrot, and green onion. Top with large chunks of fish or sliced chicken breast, if using. Serve with the Asian vegetables.

Cobb Salad

This American classic was created in the 1920s and exists in hundreds of variations. This is a quick version, but you can create your own variation using your favorite vegetables.

🕐 Prep time: **10** minutes   🕐 Total time: **10** minutes

(15 if cooking bacon)

---

4 cups torn romaine lettuce leaves
1 apple, cored and sliced
½ avocado, sliced
1 tomato, cut into 8 wedges
1 cup cooked chicken or turkey breast
2 slices cooked Canadian bacon, chopped (optional)
2 teaspoons shredded low-fat cheddar cheese or crumbled blue cheese
For the dressing
2 tablespoons nonfat or low-fat yogurt or mayonnaise
2 tablespoons apple juice
1 tablespoon balsamic vinegar
1½ teaspoons olive oil
¼ teaspoon sugar substitute
Pinch of salt
Pinch of black pepper

1. Toss the lettuce with the apple and avocado in a salad bowl and assemble on two plates. Place the tomato wedges around the sides of the plates. Top with the cooked chicken/turkey and bacon, if using. Sprinkle with the cheese.

2. Prepare the dressing by combining all the dressing ingredients in a small jar with a lid. Shake well. Serve the dressing on the side and use for dipping, or toss the dressing with the salad.

Cottage Cheese Salad

This creamy, crunchy salad can also be stuffed into a whole-wheat pita.

Prep time: **15** minutes   Total time: **15** minutes

1 cup low-fat cottage cheese
1 stalk celery, chopped
2 radishes, finely chopped
1 green onion, chopped
1 small apple, cored and chopped
1 teaspoon minced fresh ginger
1 teaspoon soy sauce
1 small clove garlic, minced
½ teaspoon rice vinegar
¼ teaspoon sesame oil

Combine all the ingredients in a medium bowl and stir well.

Super Express: Mixed Greens with Pears, Pecans and Chèvre

Prep time: **10** minutes   Total time: **15** minutes

1 or 2 ripe but firm pears
¼ cup pecan halves, toasted
2 cups prewashed mixed salad greens
1 ounce goat cheese (chèvre), crumbled
For the dressing
2 tablespoons apple juice
1 tablespoon balsamic vinegar
¼ teaspoon sugar substitute
Pinch of salt
Pinch of black pepper
1½ teaspoons olive oil

Sides Suggestions (see Basics page 50)
Canadian bacon slices
New potatoes

1. Prepare the potatoes according to the basic instructions.

2. Core the pears and cut into 8 slices.

3. Toast the pecans in a skillet placed over a medium heat for 2–3 minutes, until lightly browned.

4. Combine all the dressing ingredients except the oil in a medium bowl, then whisk in the oil. Toss the greens with the dressing. Divide the greens between 2 plates and top with the pears. Sprinkle with the goat cheese and pecans and serve with the bacon and potatoes.

Warm Lemony Roasted Vegetable Pasta Salad

Toss in some leftover roast chicken or a can of tuna or salmon for a simple lunch or dinner. You can also try out a variety of vegetable combinations.

| Prep time: **10** minutes | Total time: **30–35** minutes |

1 shallot, chopped
1 tablespoon olive oil
1 tablespoon lemon juice
1 tablespoon Dijon mustard
1 tablespoon chopped fresh herbs (choose from a mixture of thyme, rosemary, oregano, and marjoram)
¼ teaspoon salt
¼ teaspoon black pepper
1 small eggplant, quartered, then cut crosswise into ½-inch slices
1 red bell pepper, stemmed, seeded, and cut into ½-inch pieces
1 zucchini, halved and cut into ½-inch rounds
1 small red onion, cut into wedges
4 ounces shiitake mushrooms, stems discarded and caps cut into quarters
3 ounces whole-wheat penne or other similar-size pasta shape
1 tablespoon chopped fresh basil or parsley

Sides Suggestions (see Basics page 50)
Cooked chicken or fish

1. Preheat the oven to 425°F.

2. Whisk together the shallot, oil, lemon juice, mustard, herbs, salt, and pepper in a large bowl. Add the vegetables and toss to coat with the dressing. Place on a rimmed baking sheet and roast for 20–25 minutes, turning a couple of times, until the vegetables are lightly browned and tender.

3. Meanwhile, bring a large pot of salted water to a boil. Add the pasta and cook for about 8 minutes, or until *al dente*. Drain and transfer to a large bowl. Add the roasted vegetables and basil or parsley and toss well. Serve warm or at room temperature, along with the chicken or fish.

Broccoli and Cauliflower Salad

Double this recipe, add some cooked chicken, lean ham, or turkey breast, and you have lunch prepared for the next day. You can substitute any fresh herb you like for the tarragon.

Prep time: **10** minutes	Total time: **30** minutes

(including marinating time)

3 cups broccoli florets
3 cups cauliflower florets
2 tablespoons extra-virgin olive oil
4 teaspoons lemon juice
1 tablespoon Dijon mustard
1 teaspoon chopped fresh tarragon
Pinch of salt
Pinch of black pepper
½ red onion, chopped

1. Steam the broccoli and cauliflower in a steamer basket placed over simmering water for about 5 minutes, or until tender-crisp.

2. Meanwhile, whisk together the olive oil, lemon juice, mustard, tarragon, salt, and pepper in a large bowl. Add the broccoli, cauliflower, and red onion and toss to coat. Set aside to marinate for about 20 minutes before serving. It will keep, refrigerated, for up to 3 days.

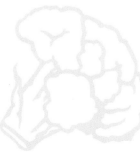

DESSERTS

Plenty of desserts are ideal for the Express G.I. Diet, as they require no preparation at all, such as:

- Fruit yogurt
- Berries with yogurt
- Cottage cheese with fruit
- ½ cup no-sugar-added ice cream

COMPANY COMING

We have included here a few recipes designed for at least four people. Most of them take only five minutes to prepare, and the rest just a few minutes longer. Enjoy.

Melon and Berries

Prep time: **5** minutes   Total time: **5** minutes

Serves 4
1 honeydew melon, cut into thin slices
2 teaspoons lime juice
1 cup blackberries
1 cup plain yogurt with sweetener (optional)

1. Place the melon in a large bowl and gently toss with the lime juice.

2. Spread the melon slices out in a fan formation over 4 plates. Sprinkle with the berries and a dollop of yogurt, if using.

Creamy Raspberry Mousse

No one will know this dessert was so easy to make. Serve it as is or dress it up with some fresh fruit or berries.

Prep time: **5** minutes   Total time: **5** minutes

Serves 4
1 cup low-fat cottage cheese
1 cup frozen raspberries
2 tablespoons sugar substitute, or to taste
1–2 teaspoons amaretto or berry-flavored liqueur (optional)

1. Combine all the ingredients in a food processor and process until smooth. Serve immediately or refrigerate in an airtight container for up to 3 days.

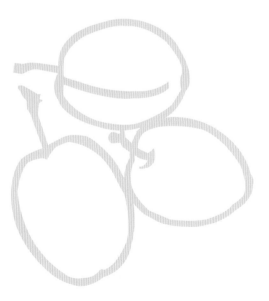

Fancy Fruit Salad

Use pretty glass serving dishes and layer the fruit for effect.
You can vary the fruit combination for color and taste.

Prep time: **10** minutes　　Total time: **10** minutes

Serves 4–6
1 pint strawberries, sliced (reserve 1 per person whole for
　garnish)
1 pint fresh berries (such as blueberries or blackberries)
1 teaspoon sugar substitute (optional)
2 tablespoons orange juice
½ teaspoon ground cinnamon
¼ teaspoon ground nutmeg
4 kiwis, peeled and sliced
Sprig of mint (optional)

1. Sprinkle the berries with sugar substitute, if using.

2. Combine together the orange juice, cinnamon, and nutmeg
in a small bowl. Layer the fruit in serving dishes, alternating
berries and kiwis and ending with slices of kiwi on top.

3. Drizzle each dish with a small amount of the orange juice
mixture. Top with a whole strawberry and mint, if using. Serve
with sweetened strained yogurt on side (see page 115).

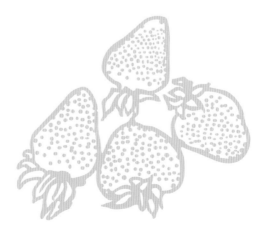

Microwave Crumble

Crumbles baked in the oven take at least 30 minutes, but by using the microwave cooking time is reduced to 5–7 minutes. The top does not become golden or crisp in the microwave, but the taste is still delicious. Try a variety of fruit combinations and adjust the sugar substitute to taste.

Prep time: **10** minutes   Total time: **16** minutes
(if using microwave)

Serves 6

3 cups fresh or frozen and thawed berries (such as blueberries and blackberries)
2 large apples, cored and chopped
2 tablespoons whole-wheat flour
1 tablespoon sugar substitute
½ teaspoon ground cinnamon
For the topping
1 cup rolled oats
¼ cup brown sugar substitute
¼ cup nonhydrogenated soft margarine, melted
½ cup chopped pecans or walnuts
1 teaspoon ground cinnamon

1. Combine the berries and apple in an 8-inch square microwaveable baking dish. Combine the flour, sugar substitute, and cinnamon. Sprinkle the mixture over the fruit and toss gently.

2. To make the topping, combine the oats, sugar substitute, margarine, pecans, and cinnamon in a medium bowl. Sprinkle the topping over the fruit mixture. Microwave on high for about 6 minutes, or until the fruit is tender. Serve as is or with a dollop of yogurt.

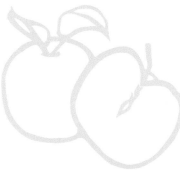

Hot Apple Slices

You can use pears in place of the apples.

Prep time: **5** minutes   Total time: **15** minutes

Serves 4
2 teaspoons nonhydrogenated margarine
4 cups sliced apples, such as Cortland or Spy
3 tablespoons sugar substitute
1 teaspoon ground cinnamon
½ teaspoon ground ginger
½ cup apple juice
½ cup water

1. Melt the margarine in a nonstick skillet over a medium-high heat. Add the apples and sprinkle with the sugar substitute, cinnamon, and ginger. Pour in the apple juice and water. Bring to a boil, then reduce the heat and simmer for 10 minutes, or until the apples have softened and the juices are syrupy.

2. Serve with a dollop of sweetened yogurt or no-sugar-added ice cream, if desired.

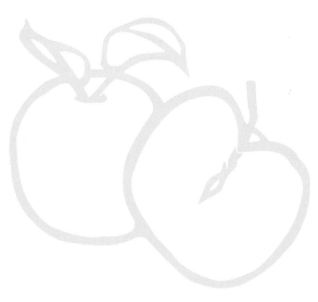

Roasted Peaches

| ⏱ Prep time: **5** minutes | 🕐 Total time: **20** minutes |

Serves 4
1 tablespoon nonhydrogenated margarine, melted
1 tablespoon sugar substitute, or to taste
½ teaspoon vanilla extract
2 fresh peaches, halved

1. Preheat the oven to 400°F.

2. Melt the margarine with the vanilla and sugar substitute in a baking dish or ovenproof skillet over a medium heat. Place the peaches cut-side-down in the baking dish, then put the dish in the oven and bake for about 15 minutes, or until the peaches are soft and the skins are starting to wrinkle.

3. Serve the peaches cut-side-up with a spoonful of low-fat ricotta or cottage cheese and drizzled with sauce from pan.

Strained yogurt

Strained yogurt with a little sweetener or some fruit spread stirred in makes a creamy addition to fresh fruit or a delicious topping for crumbles.

Place plain nonfat or low-fat yogurt in a strainer lined with cheesecloth or a coffee filter. Place the strainer over a bowl, cover with plastic wrap, and refrigerate for at least 1 hour, or overnight. Discard the liquid that drains off and transfer the yogurt to another bowl. Sweeten with sugar substitute to taste.

SNACKS

Snacks are a big part of the G.I. Diet and are even more important with the Express G.I. Diet. We recommend three snacks a day—mid-morning, mid-afternoon, and before bed. Many readers have commented that they seem to be eating all the time and are still losing weight!

Busy people frequently find themselves with little time to eat, and that's where snacks can really help. All snacks are portable and, with the exception of dairy-based foods, do not require refrigeration. From fruit, vegetables, and nuts to delicious muffins, snack bars, and scones, there are plenty of choices to keep on hand during your busy day.

"Aim to have three snacks a day."

With baked goods, such as muffins or snack bars, we recommend you make these in bulk, 12 to 24 at a time, and keep them in the freezer at home. Simply take one out when needed and microwave—or take one into the office, where they will naturally defrost. The time invested upfront will give you a dozen or so ready snacks with no additional preparation, and the results are well worth the effort.

I have grouped the snacks into two categories—ready-to-go snacks that require little or no preparation, and those with simple recipes that can be made up in bulk every couple of weeks and frozen.

The important thing to remember is to keep your tummy busy digesting food. My 96-year-old old mom likes to say, "The devil finds work for idle hands." Well, your tummy works very much along the same principle—if it's not kept busy, it starts looking for its next sugar fix!

READY-TO-GO SNACKS

There are many possible combinations of foods to give you a balanced snack. Here are some of the most popular ones:

- Fruits (fresh or frozen): apples, pears, berries, oranges, etc., with fat free yogurt and sweetener or 1% or fat free cottage cheese
- Vegetables: celery, carrots, tomatoes, cucumbers, etc., with hummus or low-fat cheese such as Laughing Cow light or Boursin light
- Fat free fruit yogurt with sweetener with a few sliced almonds
- 1% or fat free cottage cheese with a tablespoon of extra fruit jam (where fruit, not sugar, is the first ingredient listed)
- Skim milk
- Ice cream: low fat/no added sugar
- Nuts: almonds, hazelnuts, soy nuts, or macadamias (a small handful)
- Food bars: Balance Bars; Zone Bars (half a bar per serving)

RECIPES

Although these snack recipes require a bit of preparation time, you can make them in bulk batches once a month or so and store them in the freezer. They then become great timesavers, as all you have to do is slip one into the microwave for 30 seconds or take one to the office, where it will be already thawed for your mid-morning break. Try to limit yourself to one muffin or bar a day.

Muffins are unquestionably the most popular snacks, easy to make and with lots of variety. Here are a couple of delicious recipes.

Mixed Berry Muffins

Not your average bran muffin. These are moist and packed with berries.

Makes 12 muffins
1 cup All-Bran or 100% Bran cereal
1 cup wheat bran
1½ cups buttermilk
½ cup liquid egg
¼ cup canola oil
1 teaspoon vanilla extract
1 cup whole-wheat flour
½ cup sugar substitute
1 teaspoon baking soda
½ teaspoon baking powder
1½ cups mixture of blueberries and raspberries (fresh or frozen)

1. Preheat the oven to 350°F. Line or grease 12 muffin cups and set aside.

2. Combine the bran cereal and wheat bran in a large bowl. Stir in the buttermilk and set aside for 5 minutes. Stir in the egg, oil and vanilla.

3. Combine the flour, sugar substitute, baking soda, and baking powder in a separate large bowl. Stir into the bran mixture until just moistened, then stir in the berries.

4. Divide the batter among the muffin cups. Bake for about 25 minutes, or until a cake tester inserted in the center comes out clean. Remove from the oven and let the muffins cool in the pan for about 5 minutes, then remove them from the pan to a wire rack to cool slightly before serving.

Storage: The muffins can be stored, covered, at room temperature for up to 2 days or frozen for up to 1 month. To freeze, wrap each muffin individually, then place them in a resealable plastic bag or airtight container.

Orange-Cranberry Bran Muffins

The cranberries give these moist muffins a nice little burst of tartness.

Makes 12 muffins

½ cup All-Bran or 100% Bran cereal
½ cup wheat bran
1 cup buttermilk
1 omega-3 egg
¼ cup canola oil
½ cup boiling water
⅓ cup sugar substitute
1 tablespoon frozen orange juice concentrate, thawed
1 teaspoon grated orange zest
1 teaspoon vanilla extract
1 cup whole-wheat flour
¾ cup ground flaxseed
1½ teaspoons baking soda
1 teaspoon ground cinnamon
½ teaspoon ground ginger
¼ teaspoon salt
1½ cups fresh or frozen and thawed cranberries, roughly chopped

1. Preheat the oven to 400°F. Line or grease 12 muffin cups and set aside.

2. Combine the bran cereal and wheat bran in a large bowl. Stir in the boiling water to moisten and set aside for 5 minutes. Mix in the buttermilk, egg, oil, sugar substitute, orange juice concentrate, orange zest, and vanilla.

3. Combine the flour, flaxseed, baking soda, cinnamon, ginger, and salt in a separate large bowl. Stir in the cranberries. Stir into the bran mixture until just moistened.

4. Divide the batter among the muffin cups and bake for about 25 minutes, or until a cake tester inserted in the center comes out clean. Remove from the oven and let the muffins cool in the pan for about 5 minutes, then remove them from the pan to a wire rack to cool slightly before serving.

Storage: The muffins can be stored, covered, at room temperature for up to 2 days or frozen for up to 1 month. To freeze, wrap each muffin individually, then place them in a resealable plastic bag or airtight container.

BARS

Moist and chewy, these bars are a good alternative to fat- and sugar-laden commercial cereal bars. For an extra protein kick, stir in 4 tablespoons of whey or soy-protein powder with the dry ingredients.

Berry Bars

Makes 16 bars
3 cups fresh or frozen and thawed raspberries or blueberries, or a mixture of both
1 cup large flake oats
1 cup high-fiber cereal
½ cup ground flaxseed
¼ cup wheat germ
¼ cup whole-wheat flour
¼ cup sesame seeds
2 teaspoons ground cinnamon
2 egg whites
¼ cup frozen apple juice concentrate, thawed
2 teaspoons vanilla extract

1. Preheat the oven to 350°F. Grease an 8-inch square baking pan and set aside.

2. Combine the berries, oats, cereal, flaxseed, wheat germ, flour, sesame seeds, and cinnamon in a large bowl.

3. Whisk together the egg whites, apple juice concentrate, and vanilla in a medium bowl. Add to the dry mixture, stirring to thoroughly moisten.

4. Press the mixture into the baking pan and bake for 35–40 minutes, or until lightly golden and firm. Let cool in the pan completely and then cut into bars.

Storage: Place the bars in an airtight container and keep refrigerated for up to 5 days or freeze for up to 1 month.

Cran-Apple Oatmeal Bars

Makes 24 bars
3 cups rolled oats
1 ½ cups whole-wheat flour
1 teaspoon baking powder
1 teaspoon baking soda
2 teaspoons ground cinnamon
¼ teaspoon salt
¾ cup sugar substitute
¼ cup nonhydrogenated margarine
¾ cup unsweetened applesauce
1 omega-3 egg
1 egg white
2 teaspoons vanilla extract
1 cup dried cranberries

1. Preheat the oven to 350°F. Grease a 13x9-inch baking pan and line with parchment. Set aside.

2. Combine the oats, flour, baking powder, baking soda, cinnamon, and salt in a large bowl.

3. Beat together the sugar substitute and margarine in a separate bowl until fluffy. Beat in the applesauce, egg, egg white, and vanilla. Add the oat mixture and stir to combine. Stir in the cranberries. Scrape the dough into the baking pan and bake for 20 minutes, or until a cake tester inserted in the center comes out clean. Let cool in the pan completely, then cut into bars.

Storage: Place the bars in an airtight container and keep refrigerated for up to 5 days or freeze for up to 1 month.

SUMMARY—FIVE GOLDEN RULES

If you follow these five golden rules along with your green light menu, then you will lose weight painlessly, without going hungry or feeling deprived.

● **Drink a glass of water with each meal.** Always drink a glass of water with your lunch and dinner. Drink early on in the meal, as this will fill your tummy and help you feel fuller, sooner.

● **Divide your plate into three.** Visualize your plate in three sections: half the plate containing vegetables (at least two different types); one quarter protein (meat, fish, poultry, tofu); and one quarter carbohydrates (potatoes, rice, pasta).

● **Watch your serving sizes.** There are few restrictions on green light foods, especially fruit and vegetables. Nonetheless, moderation is the watchword. For exceptions, see page 14.

● **Don't rush your meals.** It can take half an hour for the brain to realize the stomach is full, so eat slowly to make sure that you don't overeat. Try to put down your fork between mouthfuls.

● **Eat three meals and three snacks every day.** Always eat three meals and three snacks daily. Breakfast is particularly important. Keep your tummy busy all day digesting green light foods.

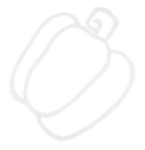

Chapter 6: Phase Two: How You Will Eat for the Rest of Your Life

Congratulations! You've reached your new weight target. You're probably feeling like a new person since you started your journey a few months ago. But be warned, you are entering a tricky stage as you shift from weight loss to weight maintenance—the phase you will maintain for the rest of your life.

This is the time when, traditionally, most people blow their diets. They have achieved their weight target, can fit into their dream dress, suit, or bikini, and so abandon their diet and return to their old eating habits. Surprise, surprise—a few months later they balloon back to where they started, or worse. Sound familiar? I bet most of my readers have experienced this at least once in their lives.

To avoid this yo-yoing, it is important to make only minor shifts in your diet and to remember that fundamental changes have taken place in your body. First, your body has become accustomed to using fewer calories than in its earlier spendthrift days. You have learned to become more energy efficient (a popular term these days with global warming!) and a body that is more efficient needs fewer calories to function.

Second, a lighter body also requires fewer calories to function than a heavy one. Just as a small car needs less fuel to run than a big one, a 160-pound person needs more calories to function than a 130-pound person. In fact, if you lose 20 pounds, you will require 250 calories less per day to function.

Your leaner and more efficient body now requires significantly fewer calories to function than when you began the program. So in shifting from losing weight to maintaining weight, you only need a modest increase in calorie consumption. Remember the equation: to maintain your weight, energy (calories) taken in has to balance energy expended.

In Phase Two we suggest you make two principal changes:

- Increase your serving sizes of green light foods by 10–20 percent, especially the ones where we listed a recommended serving size—meat, pasta, rice, bread, etc.
- Add some yellow light foods to your diet. Some popular additions are 70-percent cocoa chocolate, wine, bananas, and sirloin steak.

This will help you make the transition into the final stage of your journey. Again, moderation is the key word. If you feel yourself sliding and the weight starts to come back, you know what to do. Simply switch back to Phase One and repeat the process. This time, moderate your changes. A little trial and error is inevitable at this stage, so don't panic. You'll find the right balance very quickly.

The bottom line is that Phase Two is only marginally different from Phase One. All the fundamentals of the Phase One plan remain unbreakable. Phase Two provides an opportunity to make small adjustments to portions and add new foods from the yellow light category.

Make the most of this new-found freedom!

Chapter 7: Top Five FAQs (Frequently Asked Questions)

Out of the thousands of e-mails we've received, here are the five most popular questions, along with our responses:

Q1. I am currently on a high-protein (typically Atkins) diet and I want to change to the G.I. Diet. If I switch, will I put on some of the weight that I've struggled so hard to lose?

A.   Many diets, including the popular high-protein ones such as Atkins, are diuretics, which is one of the reasons why these diets let you lose weight so quickly in the short term. That is also one of the reasons why people want to change, as they often don't feel well or look good.

The G.I. Diet will rehydrate you, which means you may well put on a pound or two to start with, but that will be quickly lost as your new diet kicks in, providing you with a steady, healthy weight loss.

Q2. Why don't your recipes have a nutritional analysis like other diet books?

A.   One of the cornerstones of the G.I. Diet is simplicity. Rather than have you worry about nutritional analysis, counting G.I. ratings, calories, and so on, we decided to do all the analysis for you and color-code the results. Accordingly, green light recipes have a low G.I. rating and are also low in calories, sodium, and saturated fats.

Q3. I've been losing weight steadily on the G.I. Diet, but it's suddenly stopped. What should I do?

A.   Unfortunately, losing weight never occurs in a straight line. It always goes in fits and starts where you descend from one plateau to another. This occurs with women in particular because of hormonal changes in the monthly cycle.

   That is why we talk about *average* weekly weight loss in the book, as sometimes you will lose two to three pounds a week and then frequently nothing at all for a couple of weeks. So don't despair if you find yourself stuck on a plateau for a short period, as you will soon come off it and continue to lose weight. Remember, it probably took you many years to gain your current weight, so don't be impatient if it takes a few weeks longer than you anticipated to lose it.

Q4. I thought sugar substitutes were bad for your health, so why are you recommending them?

A.   Sugar substitutes or sweeteners have been approved by all the major government and health agencies worldwide as perfectly safe for your health. A great deal of disinformation has been spread by the sugar lobby in the United States, particularly on the Internet.

   Some people are sensitive to aspartame but there are many other suitable alternatives. Our particular preference is for Splenda (sucralose), which tastes like sugar, but without the calories.

Q.5. I'm feeling like a short-order cook trying to eat the green
light way while looking after the different food needs of
my husband and children. Can the whole family follow the
G.I. Diet whether they have a weight problem or not?

A.   The whole family can and should eat the green light way.
The G.I. Diet is a healthy and nutritious way to eat for the
whole family, whether they be reluctant spouses/partners,
junk-food-possessed teens, or finicky toddlers. By simply
making small adjustments to serving sizes, all the family's
nutritional needs can be met. As importantly, you will be
developing healthy eating habits for your children that
will have an impact on the eating habits of their future
families.

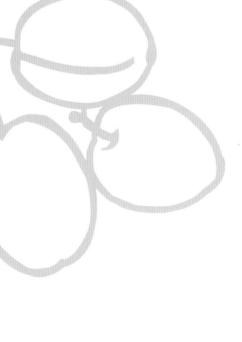

Chapter 8: Exercise

While exercise is essential for good health and weight maintenance, frankly, it is not that imperative when it comes to losing weight. To put this in perspective, have a look at the following table, which shows how much exercise you need in order to lose just 1 pound of fat.

EFFORT REQUIRED TO LOSE 1LB OF FAT

	130 pound person	160 pound person
Walking (4mph–brisk)	53 miles/85km	42 miles/67km
Running (8min/mile)	36 miles/58km	29 miles/46km
Cycling (12–14mph)	96 miles/154km	79 miles/127km
Sex (moderate effort)	79 times	64 times

Clearly, unless you are an Olympic athlete, this is not the most practical way to get those pounds off. Don't misunderstand me—any exercise will help to reduce weight, but changing your diet will have a far greater impact on helping you reach your target weight during Phase One. In the long term, if you are to maintain your weight and health, exercise is an essential component. Yet, despite good intentions, there just doesn't seem enough time in the day to devote to getting and keeping your body in shape.

The answer is to incorporate some activity into your daily routine so that it doesn't become that "added extra" that you never seem to have time for. I call this activity the "Two Stops Short" program.

TWO STOPS SHORT

As most readers have to travel from home to work, simply get off the bus or subway two stops short of your work destination. If driving, park half a mile or a mile before your usual parking spot. At the end of the day, do the reverse and get on two stops farther down the road where you disembarked in the morning. For most people this will represent about fifteen minutes' brisk walk each way. That's probably no more than ten minutes' incremental time each way compared to staying on the bus or parking closer. Maybe you'll even save a dollar or two by parking farther out!

I did this personally for several years and can vouch for the fact that the results will amaze you. If you do this year round you will use up the energy equivalent of ten pounds of fat. You will also feel healthier and more energetic and sleep better. Not a bad investment in return for just twenty extra minutes a day! This method will also afford you some peaceful thinking time in your own company. Why not try it for a couple of weeks? I promise you'll be delighted with the way you'll soon look and feel.

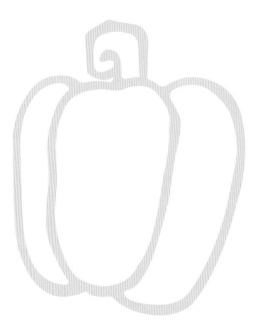

Appendix I
COMPLETE G.I. DIET FOOD

RED

BEANS

Fava (broad) beans

BEANS (CANNED)

Baked beans with pork
Refried beans

YELLOW

Kidney beans (canned)
Lentils (canned)

GREEN

BEANS

Black	Lima
Black eyed	Mung
Butter	Pigeon
Chickpeas	Pinto
Edamame (soy beans)	Romano
Haricot/Navy	Soy
Italian	Split peas
Kidney (red/white)	
Lentils	

BEANS (CANNED)

Baked beans (low-fat)
Mixed salad beans
Most varieties
Vegetarian chili

BEVERAGES

Alcoholic drinks*

Fruit drinks

Milk (whole)

Regular coffee

Regular soft drinks

Sweetened fruit juice

BEVERAGES

Diet soft drinks (caffeinated)

Milk (semi-skim)

Red wine

Diet soft drinks (no caffeine)

Unsweetened fruit juices

Vegetable juice cocktails (e.g. V8)

BEVERAGES

Bottled water

Decaffeinated coffee (with skim milk, no sugar)

Herbal teas

Light instant chocolate

Milk (skim)

Tea (with skim milk, no sugar)

Soy milk (low-fat, plain)

RED

BREADS

Bagels
Baguette/Croissants
Cereal/Granola bars
Cornbread
Crispbreads
Doughnuts
Hamburger buns
Hot dog buns
Kaiser rolls
Melba toast
Muffins
Pancakes/Waffles
Pizza
Stuffing
Tortillas
White bread

YELLOW

BREADS

Pita (wholewheat)
Wholegrain breads
Crispbread with fiber
Sourdough bread
Tortillas (low carb)

GREEN

BREADS

100% stone-ground
wholewheat*
Homemade muffins
(see p.118-9)
Wholegrain, high-fiber
breads (2½ to 3g of fiber per slice)*
Crispbreads (high-fiber) 2 per serving

*Limit portions. See p.14

CEREALS

All cold cereals
except those listed
as yellow
or green-light
Granola
Instant/quick cook oatmeal
Muesli (commercial)

CEREAL GRAINS

Almond flour
Couscous
Rice (short-grain,
white, instant)
Rice cakes
Croutons
Amaranth
Millet
Polenta
Rice noodles

CEREALS

Shredded Wheat Bran
Kashi Good Friends
Kashi Go Lean Crunch

CEREAL GRAINS

Corn
Corn flour
Spelt

CEREALS

All-Bran
Bran Buds
Fiber 1
Oat bran
Oatmeal (traditional large-flake)
100% Bran
Soy Protein Powder
Steel-cut oats
Kashi Go Lean

CEREAL GRAINS

Arrowroot flour
Barley
Buckwheat
Bulgur
Gram flour
Kamut (not puffed)
Kasha (toasted buckwheat)
Quinoa
Rice (basmati, wild, brown, long-grain)
Soy Protein Powder
Wheatgrain
Wheat berries

RED

CONDIMENTS/SEASONINGS

Croutons
Ketchup
Mayonnaise
Tartar sauce

YELLOW

Mayonnaise (light)

GREEN

CONDIMENTS/SEASONINGS

Chili powder
Extracts (Vanilla etc.)
Garlic
Herbs/Spices
Horseradish
Hummus
Lemon/lime juice
Mayonnaise (fat-free)
Lemon/lime juice
Mustard
Peppers (all types)
Salsa (low-sugar)
Soy sauce (low-sodium)
Teriyaki sauce
Vinegars (all types)
Worcestershire sauce

DAIRY

Cheese
Chocolate milk
Cottage cheese (whole/2%)
Cream
Cream cheese
Goat's milk
Milk (whole/2%)
Sour cream
Yogurt (whole/2%)
Almond milk
Rice milk
Evaporated milk

DAIRY

Cheese (low-fat)
Cream cheese (light)
Ice cream (low-fat)
Milk (1%)
(low-fat, low-sugar)
Soft margarine
(non-hydrogenated)
Sour cream (light)
Yogurt (low-fat)

DAIRY

Almond milk (low fat)
Buttermilk (skim/1%)
Cheese (fat-free)
Cottage cheese (1% or fat free)
Cream cheese (fat-free)
Frozen yogurt Fruit yogurt
(fat-free/with sweetener)
Ice cream
(low-fat and no added sugar)
Milk (skim)
Sour cream (fat-free)
Laughing Cow cheese/light
Boursin cheese/light
Soy cheese/low-fat
Soy milk (plain, low-fat)
Soy/whey protien powder

RED

FATS/OILS/DRESSINGS

Butter
Coconut oil
Hard margarine
Lard
Mayonnaise
Palm oil
Salad dressings (regular)
Tropical oils
Vegetable shortening

*Limit portions. See p14

YELLOW

FATS/OILS/DRESSINGS

Corn oil
Mayonnaise (light)
Peanut oil
Salad dressings (light)
Sesame oil
Soft margarine
(non-hydrogenated)
Soy oil
Sunflower oil
Vegetable oils

GREEN

FATS/OILS/DRESSINGS

Canola oil*
Flax seed oil*
Mayonnaise (low-fat/low sugar)
Olive oil*
Salad dressings (low-fat/low sugar)
Soft margarine (non-hydrogenated, light)*
Vegetable oil sprays
Vinaigrette

FRUITS—FRESH

Cantaloupe
Dates
Honeydew melon
Kumquats
Melons
Watermelon

FRUITS—FRESH

Apricots (fresh)
Bananas
Custard apples
Kiwi
Mangoes
Papaya
Persimmon
Pineapple
Figs

FRUITS—FRESH

Apples
Blackberries
Blueberries
Cherries
Grapefruit
Grapes
Guavas
Lemons
Limes
Oranges
Nectarines
Peaches
Pears
Plums
Raspberries
Rhubarb
Strawberries

RED

FRUITS—BOTTLED, CANNED, FROZEN, DRIED

All canned fruit in syrup
Apple sauce (sweetened)
Most dried fruit*
Raisins

*For baking, it is OK to use a modest amount of dried fruit

FRUIT SPREADS

Regular fruit spreads

FRUIT JUICES

Fruit drinks
Sweetened juices
Prune
Watermelon

YELLOW

FRUITS—BOTTLED, CANNED, FROZEN, DRIED

Dried apricots
Dried cranberries
Fruit cocktail in juice
Peaches/pears in syrup
Prunes

FRUIT JUICES

Apple (unsweetened)
Cranberry (unsweetened)
Grapefruit (unsweetened)
Orange (unsweetened)
Pear (unsweetened)
Pineapple (unsweetened)

GREEN

FRUITS—BOTTLED, CANNED, FROZEN, DRIED

Apple sauce (unsweetened)
Dried apples
Frozen berries
Mandarin oranges
Peaches in juice or water
Pears in juice or water

FRUIT SPREADS

Extra fruit/low-sugar spreads
(fruit as first ingredient)

FRUIT JUICES

Eat the fruit rather than
drink the juice

MEAT, POULTRY, FISH, EGGS AND TOFU

Bacon strips

Beef (short ribs, brisket, regular ground)

Boiled ham

Bologna (all meats)

Chicken/turkey (breast/thigh/wing with skin, Roasters/stewing light/dark with skin)

Duck

Fish and shellfish (breaded/battered)

Goose

Hamburgers

Hot dogs

Lamb (rack)

Offal

Organ meats

Pastrami (beef)

Pate

Pork (blade, back ribs, spare ribs, cured)

Regular eggs

Ground beef (more than 10% fat)

Salami

Sausages

MEAT, POULTRY, FISH, EGGS AND TOFU

Beef (sirloin tip, sirloin, T-bone, tenderloin, lean ground, flank)

Chicken/turkey (thigh without skin, roasters stewing light/dark without skin)

Corned beef

Fish and shellfish (canned in oil)

Dried beef

Lamb (fore shank, leg shank, centre cut, loin chop)

Pork (top loin, centre loin, fresh ham, shank)

Whole Omega-3 eggs

MEAT, POULTRY, FISH, EGGS AND TOFU

Beef (top round, eye round, extra lean ground)

Chicken/turkey breast without skin

Egg beaters

Egg whites

Fish/shellfish (all fresh, frozen and canned)

Ham (deli style)

Liquid eggs

Pastrami (turkey)

Pork (tenderloin, ham extra lean, Canadian bacon)

Rabbit (lean meat)

Sashimi

Smoked salmon and trout

Turkey breast (processed)

Turkey roll

TVP (textured vegetable protein e.g. Boca)

Veal (cutlet, rib roast, blade steak, shank, loin chop)

Veggie burgers

Venison

GREEN

PASTA*

Capellini
Cellophane noodles
(mung bean)
Fettuccine
Linguine
Macaroni
Penne
Rigatoni
Spaghetti
Vermicelli

PASTA SAUCES

Light sauces with
or without vegetables
(no added sugar) e.g. Healthy Choice,
Colavita, Classico

YELLOW

PASTA*

Rice noodles

PASTA SAUCES

Sauces with vegetables

RED

PASTA*

All canned pastas
Cous cous
Gnocchi
Macaroni and cheese
Noodles (tinned)
Pasta filled with
cheese or meat

Preferably wholemeal or protein-enriched pasta

PASTA SAUCES

Alfredo
Sauces with added
meat or cheese
Sauces with added
sugar

SNACKS

Bagels
Bread
Candy
Chocolates
Cookies
Biscuits
Doughnuts
French fries
Ice cream
Instant puddings
Jell-O (all varieties)
Muffins (commercial)
Peanut butter (regular and light)
Popcorn (regular)
Potato chips/Pretzels
Raisins
Rice cakes
Sorbet
Tortilla chips

SNACKS

Bananas
Dark chocolate (70% cocoa)*
Ice cream (low-fat)
Most nuts*
100% peanut butter
Popcorn (light, microwaveable)

SNACKS

Almonds*
Applesauce (unsweetened)
Canned peaches/pears in juice or water
Cashews
Cottage cheese (1% or fat-free)
Food bars (12–15g protein; 4–5g fat) e.g. Balance/Zone
Fruit yogurt (fat-free/ with sweetener)
Ice cream (low-fat and no added sugar
Hazelnuts*
Homemade muffins (see page 118)
Macadamia nuts
Most fresh fruit
Most fresh vegetables
Most seeds
Pistachios
Soy nuts*

RED

SOUPS

All cream-based soups
Canned black bean
Canned green/split pea
Pureed vegetable

SUGAR AND SWEETENERS

Corn syrup
Glucose
Honey
Molasses
Sugar (all types)

YELLOW

SOUPS

Canned chicken noodle
Canned lentil
Canned tomato

SUGAR AND SWEETENERS

Fructose
Sugar alcohols

GREEN

SOUPS

All homemade soups
made with green-light
ingredients
Chunky bean and
vegetable soups (e.g.
Healthy Request, Healthy Choice)

SUGAR AND SWEETENERS

Aspartame
Equal
Splenda
Stevia
Sugar Twin
Sweet 'N Low

VEGETABLES

French fries
Hash browns
Parsnips
Potatoes (instant)
Potatoes (mashed or baked)
Rutabagas
Turnip

VEGETABLES

Artichokes
Beets
Corn
Potatoes (boiled)
Pumpkin
Squash
Sweet potatoes
Yams

VEGETABLES

Alfalfa sprouts
Arugula
Asparagus
Avocado (per ¼ serving)
Beans (green/runner)
Bok choy
Broccoli
Brussels sprouts
Cabbage
Carrots
Cauliflower
Celery
Collard greens
Cucumber
Eggplant
Kale
Lettuce
Mushrooms
Mustard greens

Okra
Olives*
Onions
Parsley
Peas
Peppers (bell)
Peppers (chilies)
Pickles
Potatoes (new only)
Radicchio
Radishes
Sauerkraut
Snow peas
Sugar snap peas
Swiss chard
Spinach
Tomatoes
Zucchini

Appendix II: Seven-Day Meal Plan

Let the sample menu below be a guide. You can substitute other recipes and suggestions from this book. Each dinner recipe in the book is accompanied with quick side dish suggestions to enable you to get the dinner on the table in thirty minutes maximum. Enjoy.

MONDAY

BREAKFAST
Oatmeal (page 58)

SNACK
Fruit yogurt and almonds

LUNCH
Open-faced deli ham sandwich with grainy mustard and salad

SNACK
Muffin[1] (pages 118–9)

DINNER
Super-Express Oriental Salmon with Leeks (page 80)

SNACK
Fresh berries tossed in lime juice and nonfat or low-fat sour cream

TUESDAY

BREAKFAST
Muesli (page 57)

SNACK
Carrots, cucumber, sliced bell peppers with Laughing Cow low-fat cheese

LUNCH
Mixed Bean Salad (page 102)

SNACK
Apple and almonds

DINNER
Tarragon Chicken with Mushrooms (page 72)

SNACK
Canned or fresh peaches with low-fat cottage cheese

WEDNESDAY

BREAKFAST
Oatmeal (page 58)

SNACK
Berry Bars (page 120)

LUNCH
Open-faced tuna salad sandwich[2]

SNACK
BabyBel Gouda Lite (2 mini) and pear

DINNER
Speedy Pork and Lentils (page 93)

SNACK
Fancy Fruit Salad (page 112) with ½ cup low-fat, no-sugar-added
ice cream

THURSDAY

BREAKFAST
Bran-Delicious Cereal (page 57)

SNACK
Light cottage cheese with fruit

LUNCH
Cottage Cheese and Fruit (page 64)[3]

SNACK
Muffin (pages 118–119)

DINNER
Citrus Fish Steaks (page 85)

SNACK
Sliced pears with soy pudding

FRIDAY

BREAKFAST
Oatmeal (page 58)

SNACK
Light cottage cheese with fruit (page 64)

LUNCH
Open-faced deli chicken or turkey breast with grainy mustard
and salad

SNACK
Muffin (pages 118–119)

DINNER
Sautéd Greens with Ginger (page 96)

SNACK
Fruit yogurt and fresh berries

SATURDAY

BREAKFAST
Smoked Salmon Scrambled Eggs (page 60)

SNACK
Berry Bar (page 120)

LUNCH
Cobb Salad (page 115)

SNACK
Fruit and almonds

DINNER
Cocoa Spice-rubbed Grilled Steak (page 88)

SNACK
Microwave Crumble (page 113)

SUNDAY

BREAKFAST
Muesli (page 57)

SNACK
Carrots, cucumber, and sliced bell peppers with hummus

LUNCH
Mixed Greens with Pears, Pecans, and Chèvre with lean deli ham (page 117)

SNACK
Muffin (pages 118–119)

DINNER
Roasted Chicken with Tomatoes and Asparagus (page 74)

SNACK
Creamy Raspberry Mousse (page 111)

1. Make muffins and muesli bars in bulk on weekends. Wrap individually and freeze.

2. See the Lunch section on page 60 for tips on making sandwiches.

3. Why not give yourself a day off and buy lunch using the recommended lunch suggestions page 64.

Appendix III
G.I. DIET WEEKLY WEIGHT/WAIST

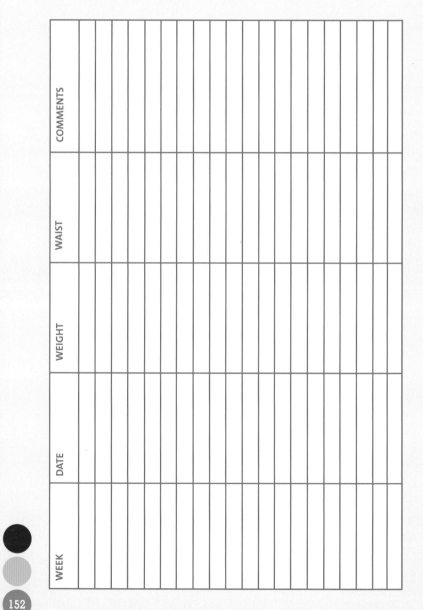

WEEK	DATE	WEIGHT	WAIST	COMMENTS	

WEEK	DATE	WEIGHT	WAIST	COMMENTS

Appendix IV: G.I. Diet Readers' Letters

If you had said to me six months ago that by Christmas I would be down to a weight similar to that of my late teens, I would never have believed you!

I purchased the first book in June and I, and many people I know, are astounded with the weight loss I have achieved. I have gone from just over 180 pounds to 140 pounds in 6 months! But the best thing is that I have not had to compromise my love of food. *Susie*

I went to the doctor and was diagnosed with Poly-Cystic Ovarian Syndrome (PCOS). My husband and I were trying to conceive without success. My doctor basically told me if I wanted to have a baby, I would need to lose weight. When I stumbled upon your G.I. Diet, I thought it was a Godsend, as if it was specifically designed for me in my time of need! After about 5—6 months, I had lost 30 pounds that were definitely staying off. Not only was I looking great, but I was feeling great. I am 3 months' pregnant expecting our first child in August! Not only did I get pregnant, but I got pregnant naturally— without fertility or blood-sugar-related drugs! It's literally a miracle. I thank God for your G.I. Diet, though I consider it more of a lifestyle than a diet. It has truly changed my life for the better! Thank you! *Erin*

My daughters bought me your book and I decided to try it, but with little thought that it would work. Anyway, just over a year later I've lost nearly 55 pounds and I can walk into any shop I like and buy whatever clothes I like. I feel like a new woman! It's incredible—I've not had so much fun since university days! I love that I can eat so well, but look so good. Everyone is amazed and so many people have bought your books on my recommendation. I have 5 kids and we all eat the same things, they are probably so much healthier now too. So a great big heartfelt thank you. The G.I. eating plan is excellent because it works and it's healthy and it's so easy. Keep up the good work.
Roberta

I am 35 and have been overweight for the past 7 years. My eldest daughter has just turned 5 and is becoming aware of body image issues, and I was extremely worried that all she got from me was "I hate my fat belly." I wanted to take the focus away from weight issues and put it onto health issues instead. Now it is, "We do this to be healthy," instead of, "We do this so we don't get fat." Well, for the past 12 weeks I have been following your G.I. diet and I have gone from 140 pounds to 120 pounds and from size 12—14 to a size 10. Other than the physical benefits, I have been overwhelmed with the psychological impact this has had on me. I now believe I deserve to look good and now invest in good clothing, skincare, and hair care. It is quite liberating. Cheers, *Brenna*

INDEX

anchovies 84
antioxidants 41
apples
  Cobb Salad 105
  Cran-Apple Oatmeal Bars 121
  Hot Apple Slices 114
  with pork 92
Apricot-Mustard Dipping Sauce
  79
artichoke hearts 95
Asian foods 34
asparagus 74, 87
Atkins diet 125
avocado 105

bacon
  Cobb Salad 105
  Spinach and Bacon Salad with
    Cranberry Vinaigrette 103
bakery 28–29
baking supplies 38–39
bananas 124
Basmati rice 53
beans and legumes 31–32, 50, 130
  chick peas 96
  Chili con Carne 91
  Mixed Bean Salad 102
beef
  and Bowties 90
  Chili con Carne 91
  Cocoa Spice-Rubbed Steak 88
  sirloin steak 124
berries
  Berry Bars 120
  Cran-Apple Oatmeal Bars 121
  Cranberry Vinaigrette 103
  Crumble 113
  Fruit Salad 112
  Melon and Berries 110

Mixed Berry Muffins 118
Orange-Cranberry Bran
  Muffins119
Raspberry Mousse 111
beverages 41, 131
Black Bean Sauce and Scallops 82
body mass index (BMI) 17–20
bran 57
  muffins 119
bread 28–29, 70, 132
breakfast 56–61, 122
  shopping 39
broccoli 109
broccoli rabe 98
brunch 61
Burger King 67

caffeine 41, 58
canned beans and vegetables
  31–32
carbohydrates 10–12
Catfish with Tomato and Cheese
  81
cauliflower 109
cereals 39, 57, 133
cheese 28, 42
  cottage cheese as snack 117
  cottage cheese and fruit 64
  Cottage Cheese Salad 106
  Mixed Greens with Pears,
    Pecans and Chèvre 107
  Raspberry and Cottage Cheese
    Mousse 111
  Tofu with Penne and Feta 101
  with catfish 81
chicken 30, 43, 53
  Chicken Fingers with Apricot-
    Mustard Dipping Sauce 79
  Chicken Peperonata 77
  Cobb Salad 105

Curried Chicken with Snow
   Peas 75
Roasted Chicken with
   Tomatoes and Asparagus 74
Sautéed Chicken Provençal 73
Sautéed Chicken with Indian
   Rice 78
Tarragon Chicken with
   Mushrooms 72
Chili con Carne 91
chocolate 124
citrus marinade 85
Cocoa Spice Rub 88, 89
coconut milk 86
cod 29
coffee 58, 71
condiments 36-37, 134
cooking techniques 46–55
Cranberry Vinaigrette 103
cucumbers 104

dairy foods 41–42, 135
desserts 70-71, 110–115
   prepared 44
dinner 71
dressings 36, 54, 63, 65, 105, 136

eating out 64–71
eggplant
   Eggplant Parmesan 99
   Roasted Vegetable Pasta Salad
     108
   Vegetable Ragout 100
eggs 42, 139
   omelets 59–60
   scrambled 59, 60–61
exercise 128–129

fast food 65–69
fats 13, 136
Fettucine with Tofu and Broccoli
   Rabe 98
fish 80–87, 139
   cooking methods 50–51

shopping 29–30
flavanoids (antioxidants) 41
frozen foods 43–44, 45
fruit 50, 137
   cottage cheese and fruit 64
   crumble 113
   dried 38, 138
   frozen 44, 51, 138
   Fruit Salad 112
   Hot Apple Slices 114
   Roasted Peaches 115
   shopping 27
   snacks 117

garlic 52
G.I. Diet
   color coding 13–14, 125
   family meals 127
   Golden Rules 122
   phases 16
ginger 94, 96
glucose 10
Glycemic Index (G.I.) 10
grains 33-34, 52
Greens Sautéed with Ginger 96
grilling, vegetables 55

halibut
   Braised 83
   Sautéed with Tomatoes and
     Anchovies 84
herbs 52, 73
high-protein diets 125

insulin 11–12

jams 40
juices 41

kitchen equipment 48–49
kiwis 112

leeks 80
lentils and pork 93

lunch 61–71

marinade, citrus 85
marlin 85
McDonald's 66-67
meals per day 15
meat 70, 139
    processed 28
Melon and Berries 110
Mexican foods 35
microwave cooking 25, 48, 113
Middle Eastern foods 35
milk 41, 42, 117
monounsaturated fats 13
muesli 57
Muffins
    Mixed Berry 118
    Orange-Cranberry Bran 119
mushrooms 72, 95
    shiitake 108
mustard 79

nutritional analysis 125
nutritional labels 22–23
nuts 13, 117
    pecans 107

oatmeal 40, 58
oils 35, 136
omega-3 oils 13, 29
omelets 59–60
Orange-Cranberry Bran
    Muffins119

pasta 32-33, 47, 52, 140
    Bowties with beef 90
    Creamy Garlic Fettucine with
        Tofu and Broccoli Rabe 98
    Noodle Salad with Cucumbers
        and Sesame Seeds 104
    Roasted Vegetable Pasta Salad
        108
    salad 62–63
    Tofu with Penne and Feta 101

Peaches, Roasted 115
pears
    Mixed Greens with Pears,
        Pecans and Chèvre 107
    with Pork Chops 94
pecan nuts 107
pickles 35
Pizza Hut 69
pork
    Chops with Pear and Ginger 94
    with Lentils 93
    Tenderloin with Apple and
        Rosemary 92
portions 15, 47, 122, 124
potatoes 25, 52, 87
poultry 53, 70, 139
prepared foods 43
proteins 12

Quinoa Salad, Curried 97

raisins 100
Raspberry Mousse 111
rice 33-34, 47, 53, 78
rosemary 92

salads 47, 53-54, 62–64, 70,
    102–109
    Broccoli and Cauliflower Salad
        109
    Cobb Salad 105
    Cottage Cheese Salad 106
    Curried Quinoa Salad 97
    dressings 36, 54, 63, 65, 105
    Mixed Bean Salad 102
    Mixed Greens with Pears,
        Pecans and Chèvre 107
    Noodle Salad with Cucumbers
        and Sesame Seeds 104
    Roasted Vegetable Pasta Salad
        108
    Salmon, Red Potato and
        Asparagus Salad 87
    Spinach and Bacon with

Cranberry Vinaigrette 103
salmon 29
    Oriental Salmon with Leeks 80
    smoked with scrambled eggs
        60–61
    with Red Potato and Asparagus
        Salad 87
salt 65
sandwiches 62, 64-65
saturated fats 13, 28, 30, 41
sauces 33, 36, 70, 82, 140
    Apricot-Mustard Dipping Sauce
        79
Scallops in Black Bean Sauce 82
seafood 43, 50–51, 70, 86
sesame seeds 104
shark 85
shopping 22, 24–45
Shrimp with Coconut Curry 86
side dishes 47
smoothies 58
snacks 37–38, 116–121, 141
snow peas 75
soups 69, 142
    shopping 33
soy 139
soy milk 41, 42
spices and flavorings 38-39, 52
spinach 103
Splenda 38, 46–47, 54, 126
steaming 55
stir-fries 55, 76, 82
strawberries 112
Subway 65-66
sugar (carbohydrates) 10–12,
        46–47, 54, 142
sweeteners 38, 54, 126, 142

Taco Bell 68
tarragon 72
tea 41, 58
tofu 30
    Fettucine with Tofu and
        Broccoli Rabe 98

with Penne and Feta 101
tomatoes 74, 81, 84
traffic light system 13–14
tuna 85
turkey 30
TVP (textured vegetable protein)
        30

Veal Piccata 95
vegetables 70, 143
    cooking 54–55
    frozen 43
    Roasted Vegetable Pasta Salad
        108
    shopping 24–26, 31–32
    snacks 117
    Vegetable Ragout with Spices
        100
vinaigrette 63, 87
    Cranberry Vinaigrette 103

waist measurement 20
waist-to-hip measurement 20–21
water 41, 70, 122
weight-loss
    maintenance 123–124
target 17–21, 123
timeline 21
uneven 126
Wendy's 67–68
Whitefish, braised 83
whole-wheat flour 28-29
wine 124

yogurt 42, 58, 115, 117